Mayara Christina Monteiro
Ana Caroline Melo de Sousa
Bianca Alves Silva

The difficulties faced by women with breast cancer

Mayara Christina Monteiro
Ana Caroline Melo de Sousa
Bianca Alves Silva

The difficulties faced by women with breast cancer

The struggle to overcome

ScienciaScripts

Imprint
Any brand names and product names mentioned in this book are subject to trademark, brand or patent protection and are trademarks or registered trademarks of their respective holders. The use of brand names, product names, common names, trade names, product descriptions etc. even without a particular marking in this work is in no way to be construed to mean that such names may be regarded as unrestricted in respect of trademark and brand protection legislation and could thus be used by anyone.

Cover image: www.ingimage.com

This book is a translation from the original published under ISBN 978-613-9-70205-3.

Publisher:
Sciencia Scripts
is a trademark of
Dodo Books Indian Ocean Ltd. and OmniScriptum S.R.L publishing group

120 High Road, East Finchley, London, N2 9ED, United Kingdom
Str. Armeneasca 28/1, office 1, Chisinau MD-2012, Republic of Moldova, Europe
Printed at: see last page
ISBN: 978-620-8-17545-0

SUMMARY

CHAPTER 1	5
CHAPTER 2	11
CHAPTER 3	28
CHAPTER 4	42
CHAPTER 5	50

DEDICATORY

This book is dedicated to my dear mum and stepdad, who have always supported me. They made me into a person of integrity, dedication and character. If I'm here today it's thanks to you, you're my inspiration.

ACKNOWLEDGEMENTS

First of all, I thank God for always keeping me firm when I thought about giving up on realising my dreams, who was my safe haven when I thought everything was going to fall apart in my life. He has always been the one who has helped me through all the moments of joy and sadness, and it is thanks to his goodness and generosity that I have the opportunity to write this book today.

I'm writing a special thank you to my family who have always been by my side telling me that I could be anything I wanted to be, thank you for being my fans.

Thank you to my friends, who put up with my stressful moments, who supported me and helped me when I needed it.

I would like to thank Professor Dr Soraya El Hakim who taught me things I never imagined I would learn, who showed me that teachers are much more than those who transmit knowledge, they are friends to keep for a lifetime.

And finally, my thanks go to you, dear reader, who took an interest in this book. I hope it really brings you knowledge and improves your understanding of the subject.

SUMMARY

Breast cancer is the most common type of cancer among women. From diagnosis to post-treatment, physical and psychological changes occur, influencing women's quality of life. An integrative review was carried out using the following descriptors: Mastectomy; Breast Cancer and Women's Health. The results of the related studies constituted three themes that identified the significance of treatment and mastectomy in women's lives. The themes identified were: Body image and sex life; Quality of life after mastectomy; Assistance and care for patients; Family during the breast cancer process; Rights of breast cancer patients. Body image is related to how women see themselves during and after breast cancer. Quality of life can be influenced by the type of surgery, the longer the surgery, the greater the difficulties in upper limb functionality, and the greater the morbidity, the more damage to general health, physical, functional, cognitive and social functions. Care must be provided in a comprehensive manner, with multi-professional support, support from family and friends, and above all support from the patient. The family needs a very special view during this process so that they can understand all the stages of the illness that their loved one is undergoing at the time. With regard to the rights and laws that ensure the entire process of the disease. The woman who has undergone treatment and mastectomy has to understand that it was a procedure so that she could have the opportunity to live longer.

Keywords: *Breast cancer; Body image; Quality of life; Care; Women.*

CHAPTER 1

INTRODUCTION

Cancer is one of the world's leading causes of death (MAJEWSKI *et a!, 2012).* It is seen by society as an irreversible process that brings with it countless meanings (MOURA *et a!,* 2010). Breast cancer affects both men and women, but is rarer in males and occurs in both developing and developed countries (FARIA *et al.,* 2016).

When it comes to women, breast cancer is the most common cancer affecting women, and it is therefore greatly feared by them, as treatment can cause both physical and psychological changes, since the breast is an icon of femininity and sexuality for women, directly affecting their quality of life (ALMEIDA, 2006; BOING *et al.,* 2017; MACHADO; SOARES; OLIVEIRA, 2017).

Therefore, choosing the treatment that is ideal for the woman is of paramount importance, where she should be instructed by a health professional who is able to offer the appropriate support, trying to resolve any doubts she may have, because the support she receives from the professional and also from her family at this time is very important. The prognosis for breast cancer is good when diagnosed early, but mortality rates are still high because diagnosis is still late due to the limitations of health services (FARIA *et al.,* 2016).

Therefore, the aim of this work is to analyse through the literature how women see themselves after breast cancer treatment and how they identify themselves after undergoing the mastectomy procedure.

METHODOLOGY

This is an integrative review, which includes the analysis of relevant research that supports decision-making and the improvement of clinical practice. It is a type of research based on material that has already been prepared, mainly consisting of books and scientific articles (MENDES; SILVEIRA; GALVÃO, 2008).

In order to carry out this article, a guiding question or hypothesis was formulated to define the study's inclusion and exclusion criteria. Through this research, the answer was: What is it like for women to accept themselves after breast cancer treatment? And how does she feel when the only solution is to have a mastectomy?

The articles must meet the following inclusion criteria for the integrative review: Address the topic of mastectomy and breast cancer in women, articles published in Portuguese, English and/or Spanish, from the last eleven years (2006 to 2017), they must be freely available online and free of charge and complete. Articles that do not meet the inclusion criteria will be excluded.

Data collection took place between August and November 2017. The bibliographic data collection was adopted from the Virtual Health Library (VHL), using the electronic databases: Scientific Electronic Library Online (SCIELO), Latin American and Caribbean Literature in Health Sciences (LILACS), in order to gather specific information relevant to carrying out the research and reliability of the data contained in the journals. The descriptors chosen were: Mastectomy; Breast Cancer and Women's Health. In this way, it is considered that the aim of this article can be achieved.

With the descriptor Mastectomy: The VHL has a total of 28,092 articles, of which 9521 are complete articles, in Brazil 122 articles, in Spain 497 articles, in Cuba 71 articles, in Portuguese 1027 articles and in Spanish 1411 articles. In LILACS there were 1349 articles, 520 of them complete, 692 articles in Portuguese and 583 articles in Spanish. SCIELO found 330 complete articles, 145 in Portuguese and 153 in Spanish.

With the descriptor Breast Cancer: In the BVS 400,107 articles, of which 162,030 were full-text articles, 14,308 in Portuguese and 19,005 in Spanish. In LILACS, 15,970 articles were found, 7373 of which were full-text articles, 7556 in Portuguese and 7042 in Spanish. SCIELO found 2,399 full articles, 892 in Portuguese and 1,106 in Spanish.

With the descriptor Women's Health: a total of 30,887 full articles were found in the BVS, 10,122 in Portuguese and 5,430 in Spanish. In LILACS, a total of 8,662 articles were found, 4707 full articles, 5690 in Portuguese and 2333 in Spanish. SCIELO found a total of 2,598 articles, 2,268 in Portuguese and 163 in Spanish.

WHAT IS CANCER?

The word cancer comes from the Greek *KARKÍNOS,* meaning crab, and was first used by Hippocrates. It is not a new pathology, as it has already been detected in Egyptian mummies dating back more than 3,000 years before Christ (BRASIL, 2011).

Nowadays, more than a hundred pathologies are called cancer, where there is a disordered growth of cells and they end up invading neighbouring organs. Normal cells multiply as a continuous process, but the disordered growth of some cells is different; instead of dying, cancer cells continue the growth process and multiply abnormally (BRASIL, 2011).

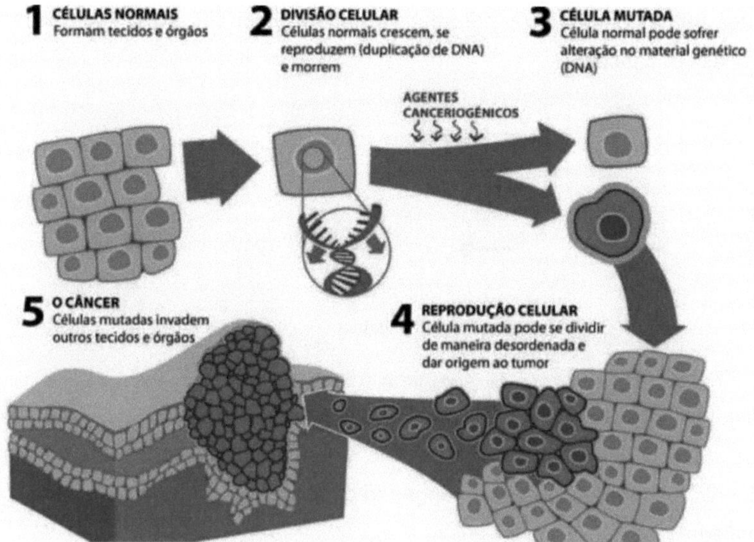

Figura 1: Cancer Cells

Source: < https://www.tuasaude.com/como-surge-o-cancer/>. Accessed on 03/08/2018.

Cell proliferation can be controlled or uncontrolled. Controlled proliferation is a localised, self-limiting increase in cells, which are normal or have minor changes in their formation and function, which may or may not be the same or different from the tissue in which they are installed. For this type of proliferation, it is normal to find hyperplasia, metaplasia and dysplasia (BRASIL, 2011).

Uncontrolled growth, on the other hand, is the abnormal and autonomous multiplication of cells. Neoplasms such as cancer in situ and invasive cancer are a type of uncontrolled growth and are considered to be tumours.

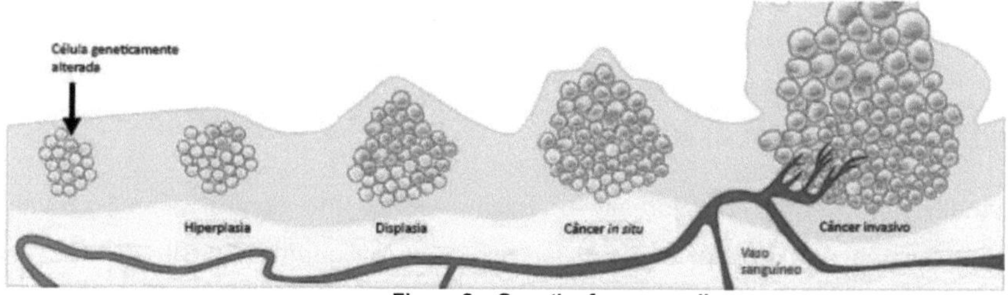

Figura 2: Growth of cancer cells

Source: Brazil. INCA, 2011.

ONCOGENESIS

As already mentioned, cells can form in a normal process where they are born and die, i.e. a mother cell creates daughter cells. However, an error can occur during this process and the daughter cell becomes totally different from the mother cell, which can start the pathological process of cancer.

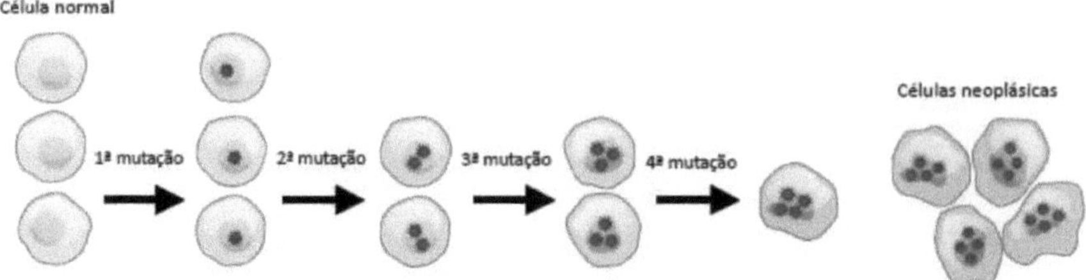

Figura 3: Cell mutation

Source: Brazil, INCA. 2011.

According to Brasil (2011), cancer goes through several stages:

- *Initiation stage:* The initial stage of cancer causes cells to suffer the effects of carcinogenic pathogens, causing changes to genes, but malignant cells cannot yet be identified;
- *Promotion stage:* The cells become malignant due to constant contact with the carcinogenic pathogen, thus creating a tumour that grows in size;
- *Progression stage:* This is the stage where multiplication is disorganised and the person with cancer begins to show signs and symptoms.

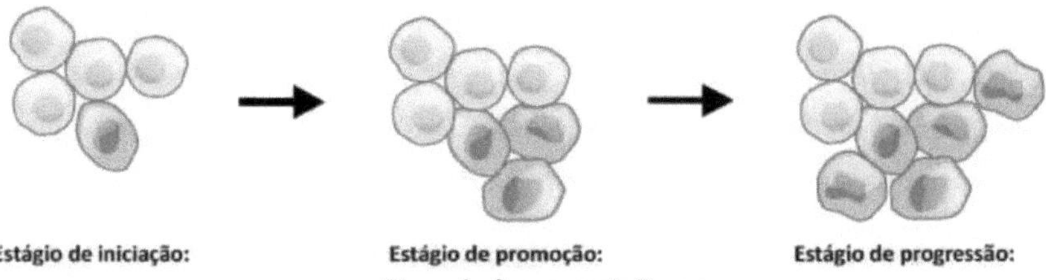

Figura 4: Oncogenesis Process

Source: Brazil, INCA. 2011.

CLASSIFICATION OF NEOPLASMS

Normally, neoplasms can partially or totally escape the control of cell growth. However, this uncontrolled growth can be called benign or malignant (BRASIL, 2011).

- *Benign neoplasms:* These can also be called benign tumours. They grow in an organised manner, are usually slow, expansive and their boundaries are visible. Although they don't invade neighbouring tissues, they end up compressing adjacent organs and tissues. Within this classification we have liponoma, which originates in fatty tissue; myoma, which originates in muscle tissue; adenoma, which originates from benign tumours in the glands (Brasil, 2011).

- *Malignant neoplasms:* known as malignant tumours, they manifest themselves autonomously and invade neighbouring tissues. They are capable of causing metastases, are very resistant and can cause death.

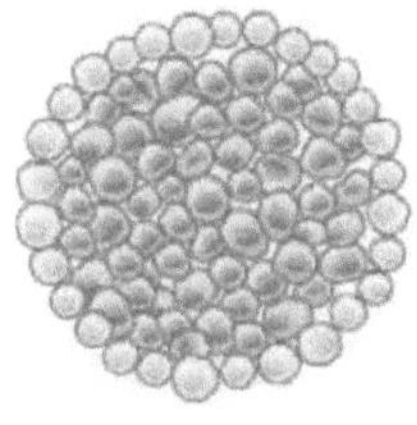

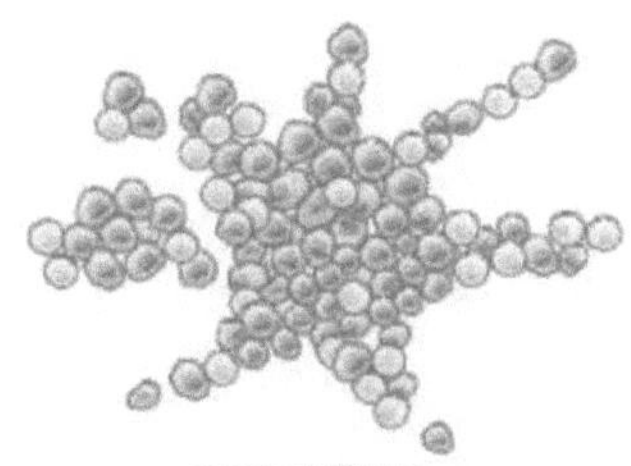

Figura 5: Difference between Neoplasms

Source: Brazil, INCA. 2011.

DIFFERENCES BETWEEN BENIGN AND MALIGNANT NEOPLASMS

Within neoplasms there are always the main differences so that you can determine what the pathology really is and the degree to which it will damage the health of its host. The main differences between benign and malignant neoplasms according to Brasil (2011) can be seen in the table below:

TABLE 1: Differences between neoplasms

BENIGN TUMOURS	*MALIGNANT TUMOURS*
Formed by well-differentiated cells (similar to those of normal tissue); typical structure of the tissue of origin.	Formed by anaplastic cells (different from those of normal tissue); atypical; lacks differentiation.
Progressive growth; may regress; normal and rare mitoses.	Rapid growth; abnormal and numerous mitoses.
Well-defined, expansive mass; does not invade or infiltrate adjacent tissues.	Poorly delimited mass, locally invasive; infiltrates adjacent tissues.
No metastasis occurs.	Metastasis often present.

Source: Brazil, INCA. 2011.

anatomy of the breast

The breast is made up of a mammary gland, which is a pair of organs located on the anterior wall of the chest, in the upper part and overlapping the pectoralis major muscle, extending from the second to the sixth rib in the vertical plane and from the sternum to the anterior axillary line in the horizontal plane (ONCOGUIA, 2014).

The female breast is made up of two lobes that give rise to milk production, ducts (small tubes that carry milk to the nipple) and stroma, which is the fatty tissue and connective tissue that surrounds the ducts and lobes, blood vessels and lymphatics

(ONCOGUIA, 2014).

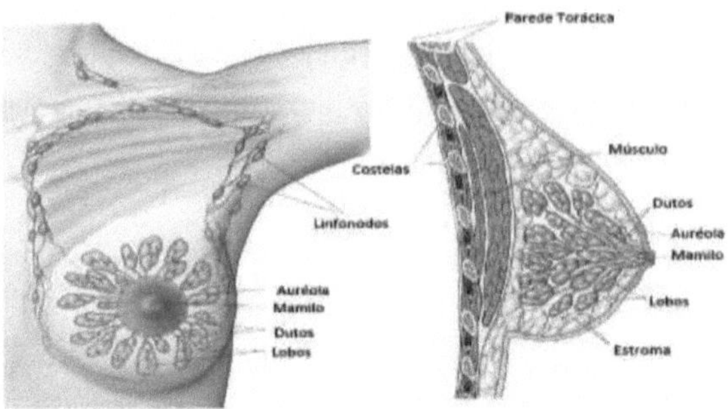

Breast anatomy.

Source: < http://www.oncoguia.org.br/conteudo/a-mama/748/12/>. Accessed on: 03/08/2018.

CHAPTER 2

FEMALE BREAST CANCER

Female breast cancer is one of the main causes of death in women in Brazil and second only to lung cancer worldwide, making it a major public health problem worldwide. It is a silent disease that is rare before the age of 35, but there are studies and references that the pathology has been affecting a considerable number of younger women in recent years (SILVA, RIUL, 2012).

The disease is one of the most frightening for women due to the great impact it has both physically and psychologically, such as: excessive anxiety, low self-esteem, acceptance of the post-mastectomy body, among others (SILVA, RIUL, 2012).

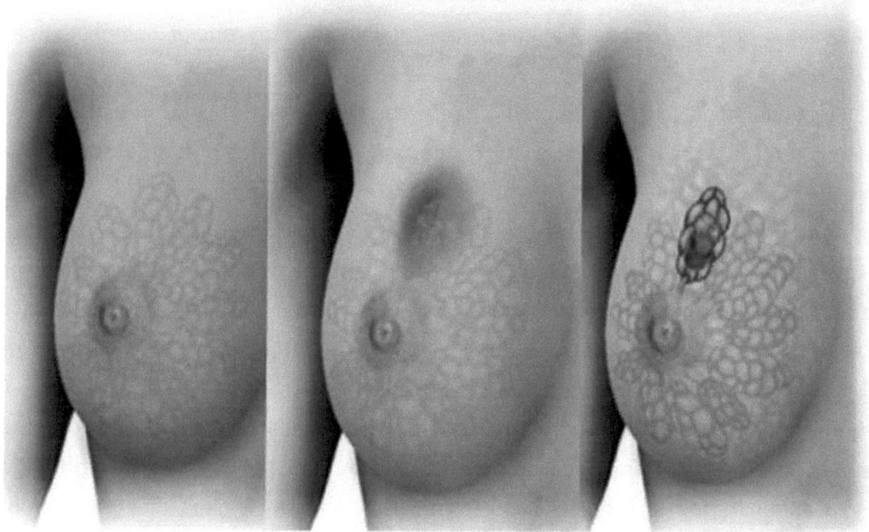

Figura 6: Breast tumour

Source: <http://emagrecer.eco.br/saude/doenca/cancer/de-mama/>. Accessed on: 03/08/2018.

When the pathology is discovered, the woman is extremely shaken because the breasts, as well as being a sexual organ, give rise to sexual differentiation, pleasure and are also completely linked to motherhood because they are the baby's source of nourishment (RAMOS; LUSTOSA, 2009).

A woman's chances of getting breast cancer are closely linked to her family history, lifestyle habits and environmental influences. With regard to family history, cancer is more common in first-degree relatives such as mothers, brothers and daughters, and the likelihood doubles with this factor. Studies also show that having two relatives with the disease increases the likelihood threefold. Life habits are defining factors for women who are obese due to the increase in oestrogen produced in adipose tissue and the climacteric period, and there are also studies which say that smoking is an influencing factor, but this is still controversial. The main environmental factor is previous exposure to ionising radiation (SILVA; RIUL, 2012).

Regarding how to discover the disease, the safest means are clinical breast examinations (CBE) and mammography. Another important test is breast self-examination, but it shows the pathology at a more advanced stage (SILVA; RIUL, 2012).

When the pathology is diagnosed, it is essential to carry out complementary diagnostic tests to determine the stage of the neoplasm according to the TNM system so that the most harmonious choice of breast cancer treatment can be made. Treatment involves partial or total removal, chemotherapy, immunotherapy and/or homonotherapy (RIBEIRO, 2014).

It is understood that female breast cancer is a malignant neoplasm, which is the disordered growth of cells causing the formation of malignant tumours, the changes in women are nodules in the breast, which may or may not be accompanied by pain in the breast or in the breast is very related to changes in breast size and shape or increased thickness of a certain part of the breasts, there may also be the outflow of blood or retraction of the nipples, already in the arms to identify it is necessary the appearance of a nodule and / or a swelling in the axillary region (RAMOS; LUSTOSA, 2012).

As far as the patient's psychological state is concerned, it will be very fragile, because society's prejudice against the condition means that many patients try to keep their illness a secret until signs show. Family feelings are sometimes positive, such as caring for the patient, but often the feeling is one of exclusion and limitation, causing the patient to develop another pathology, such as depression, which will cause her to become isolated, feel ashamed and further aggravate her condition (RAMOS; LUSTOSA, 2012).

What is also of great importance is the dynamics and how the doctor and the health team will deal with this patient, thus bringing emotional support, a comfort to be making her feel at ease and creating a bond of trust between patient and health team, because when there is no such link there can be greater wear and tear on the treatment thus reducing the process of improvement (RAMOS; LUSTOSA, 2012).

TYPE OF BREAST CANCER

- *Non-invasive:* Non-invasive female breast cancer is also called in situ cancer, which is cancer that is confined to some part of the breast, without spreading to other organs. The membrane covering the tumour doesn't tear and the cancer cells remain attached to the nodule.

- *Invasive:* Invasive breast cancer occurs when this same membrane is ruptured and the cancerous cells take over other parts of the body. All in situ cancer has the capacity to become invasive.

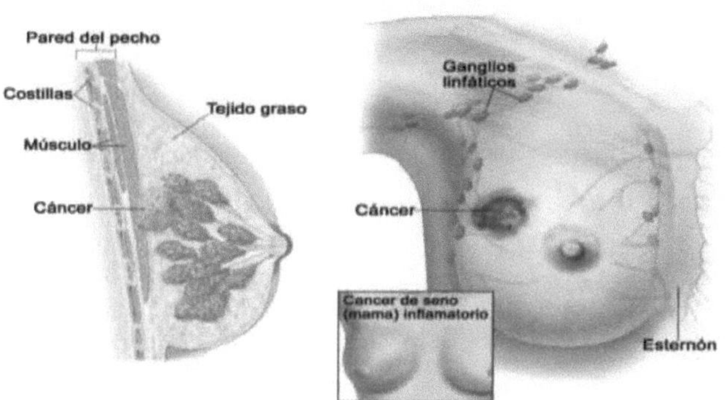

Figura 8: Types of Cancer.
Source: <https://viviendolasalud.com/enfermedades/cancer-mama>. Accessed on 03/08/2018.

SYMPTOMS OF THE DISEASE

According to INCA (2018) the pathology can be discovered in the early stages, most often by early signs and symptoms such as:

- A nodule, a swelling (lump), which is physical and most often painless, is the main manifestation of the pathology and is present in around 90 per cent of cases when the disease is noticed by the patient herself.

-Breasts retracted, with reddened skin or an orange peel appearance.

-Small nodules in the armpits and neck.

-Alteration of the nipple.

-Abnormal discharge of fluid from the breasts.

The symptoms mentioned should always be investigated, but the disease can be benign. It is important for women to always have another examination and to know what is normal in their bodies, because if there are any changes, it will be easier to uncover not only an abnormality in the breasts but also in any other area of the body (INCA, 2018).

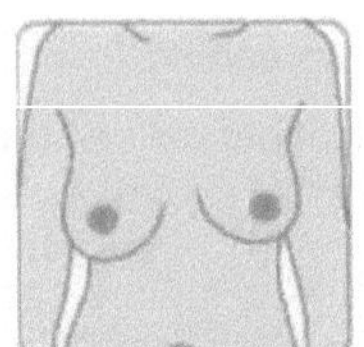

Alteração no tamanho ou na forma da mama

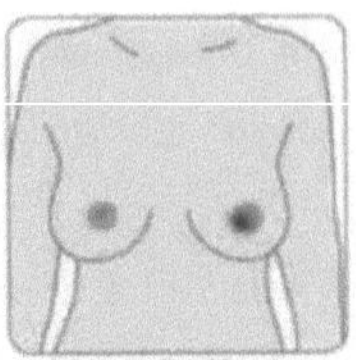

Vermelhidão ou coceira na mama e/ou ao redor do mamilo

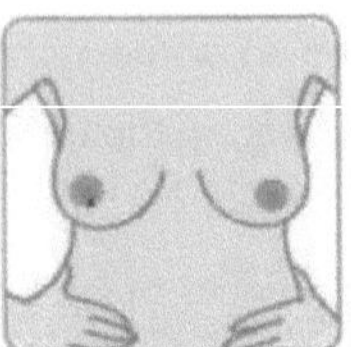

Liberação de líquido pelo mamilo, sem apertar

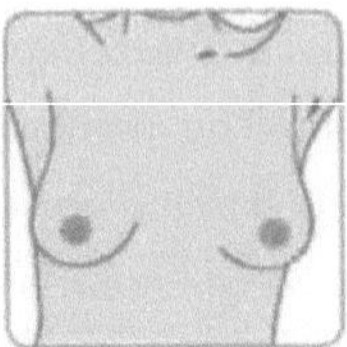

Inchaço na axila ou ao redor da clavícula

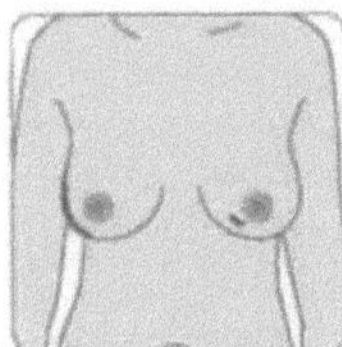

Nódulo ou caroço na mama, que está sempre presente e não diminui de tamanho

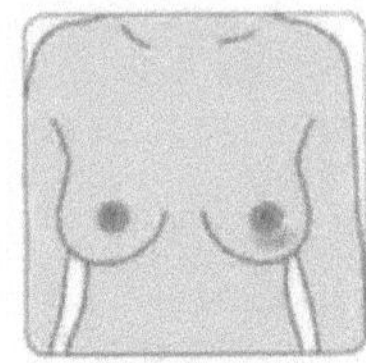

Afundamento da mama, endurecimento ou enrugamento da pele (casca de laranja)

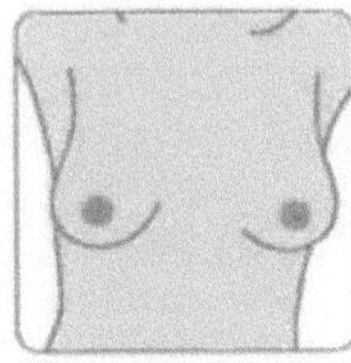

Inversão súbita do mamilo

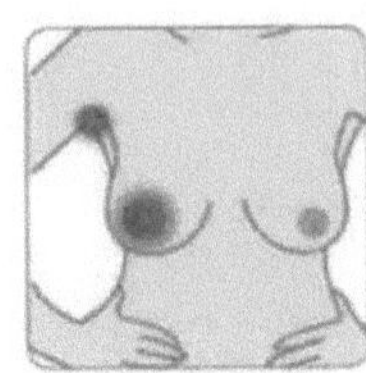

Dor constante na mama ou na axila

Figure 9: Symptoms of Breast Cancer

Source: < http://www.imeb.com.br/12-sintomas-do-cancer-de-mama/ >. Accessed on 09/08/2018.

BREAST CANCER STAGING

Staging is the definition and assessment of the anatomical extent of the cancer in the human body, i.e. how far the cancer has progressed through the body, and is divided as follows (XAVIER, 2009):

- Stage 1: The cancer cells are still contained, at this stage it is always curable;
- Stage 2: The tumour is already at least 2 cm, but has not yet advanced to the axillary glands;
- Stage 3: The tumour is over 5 cm, may or may not have advanced into neighbouring tissues, but there is no evidence that it is in the process of metastasising.
- Stage 4: The tumours can be any size, in the vast majority of cases they have already reached the lymph glands.

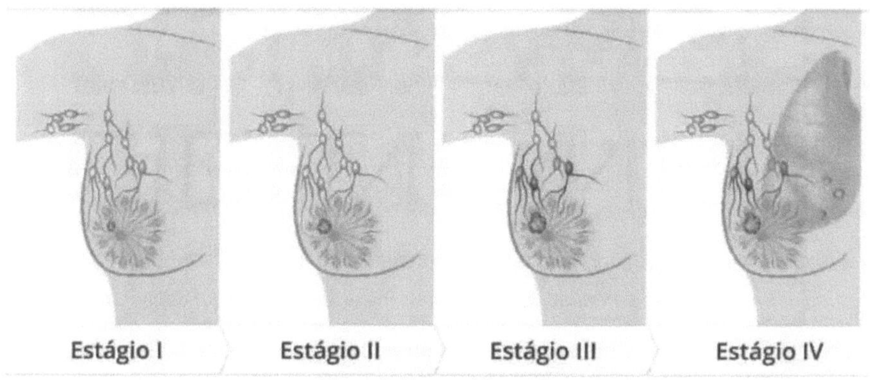

Figure 0: Stages of Breast Cancer

Source: <http://zedudu.com.br/sespa-lana-campanha-outubro-rosa-para-combater-o-cncer-de-mama/>. Accessed on: 31/07/2018.

Between the 1940s and 1950s, a staging system called TNM was developed, which was later adopted as the only system for classifying the progress of cancer. The TNM system works in the form of a three-component survey, where T is the extent of the primary tumour; N is the absence or presence of metastasis in regional lymph nodes and M is the absence or presence of distant metastasis (XAVIER, 2009).

In order to carry out the assessment correctly, all the components must be realised, as can be seen below:

- *Anatomical sub-regions.*
- *Definition of regional lymph nodes.*
- *TNM - Clinical Classification - Tumour / Nodule / Metastasis.*
- *pTNM - Pathological Classification*
- *G - Histopathological grading*
- *Rating R*
- *Grouping by stadium*
- *Schematic summary*

There are two classifications for the anatomical site, one clinical and the other histopathological (Xavier, 2009). Within the clinical classification, TNM or cTNM assessments are made, so that the therapeutic approach can be defined. The histopathological classification is only carried out after biopsy surgery and is essential for determining the prognosis (Xavier, 2009).

The lymph nodes that are examined are the lymph nodes and the axillary lymph nodes, which are divided as follows according to Xavier (2009):

- *Level I or lower axillary: lymph nodes located externally to the lateral edge of the pectoralis minor muscle.*

- *Level II or middle axillary: lymph nodes situated between the medial and lateral borders of the pectoralis minor muscle and the interpeitorial or Rotter's lymph nodes.*

- *Level III or upper axillary: lymph nodes located within the medial border of the pectoralis minor muscle, including the so-called subclavicular, infraclavicular or apical lymph nodes.*

The internal mammary nodes are the lymph nodes located in the intercostal spaces along the edge of the sternum (XAVIER, 2009). The regional lymph nodes are assessed as follows (XAVIER, 2009):

- *NX: regional lymph nodes cannot be assessed.*

- *N0: no metastasis in regional lymph nodes.*

- *N1: metastasis in axillary lymph node, homolateral, mobile.*

- *N2: metastasis in axillary lymph nodes attached to each other or to other structures.*

- *N3: metastasis in the lymph node of the homolateral internal mammary chain.*

In general, the following definitions are used for the systematic classification of breast tumours (XAVIER, 2009):

- *TX: primary tumour cannot be assessed.*

- *TO: no evidence of primary tumour.*

- *Tis: carcinoma in situ (intraductal Ca or lobular Ca in situ, or Paget's disease of the nipple without tumour).*

- *T1: tumour greater than or equal to 2 cm in its largest dimension.*

- *T1a: less than or equal to 0.5cm in its greatest dimension.*

- *T1b: larger than 0.5cm and smaller than 1cm in its largest dimension.*

- *T1c: larger than 1cm and smaller than 2cm in its largest dimension.*

- *T2: tumour larger than 2cm and smaller than 5cm in its largest dimension.*

- *T3: tumour larger than 5cm in its greatest dimension.*

- *T4: tumour of any size with direct extension to the chest wall or skin.*

- *T4a: extension to the chest wall.*

- *T4b: oedema or ulceration of the breast skin, or presence of satellite skin nodules confined to the same breast.*

- *T4c: T4a and T4b together.*

- *T4d: inflammatory carcinoma.*

Another definition used and fundamental to the TNM system is the notification of metastasis (XAVIER, 2009):

- *MX: presence of distant metastasis cannot be assessed.*

- *MO: no distant metastasis.*

- *M1 distant metastasis.*

- category M1 can be further specified according to the following annotations (XAVIER, 2009):

- *Pulmonary: PUL.*

- *Bone; OSS.*

- *Hepatic: HEP.*

- *Brain: CER.*

- *Lymph node: LIN.*

- *Bone marrow: MO.*

- *Pleural: PLE.*

- *Peritoneal: PER.*

- *Suprarenal: ADR.*

- *Skin: CUT.*

- *Other: OUT.*

MALE BREAST CANCER

Breast cancer is most talked about and cited in relation to women, but it can also affect men, as it develops in cells that are also located in male nipples *(AMERICAN CANCER SOCIETY, 2017).*

The pathology is most common in men aged between 50 and 65 and the disease may be more favourable for men who already have a family history of *breast* cancer *(AMERICAN CANCER SOCIETY, 2017).*

It is important to know that the use of anabolic steroids or oestrogen can increase the possibility of breast cancer developing in men. Other risks include radiation, cirrhosis and alcoholism, which can be more conducive to the development of the disease *(AMERICAN CANCER SOCIETY, 2017).*

The possible signs and symptoms of male breast cancer are as follows:

-Lump or swelling, usually painless.

-Wrinkled or wavy skin.

-Nipple retraction.

-Swelling in the lymph nodes.

-Redness or peeling of the breast or nipple.

These changes are not always caused by cancer. One example is that most breast lumps in men are caused by gynaecomastia. Therefore, if you or someone you know has any abnormal changes in their breasts, consult a doctor so that an effective diagnosis can be made *(AMERICAN CANCER SOCIETY, 2017).*

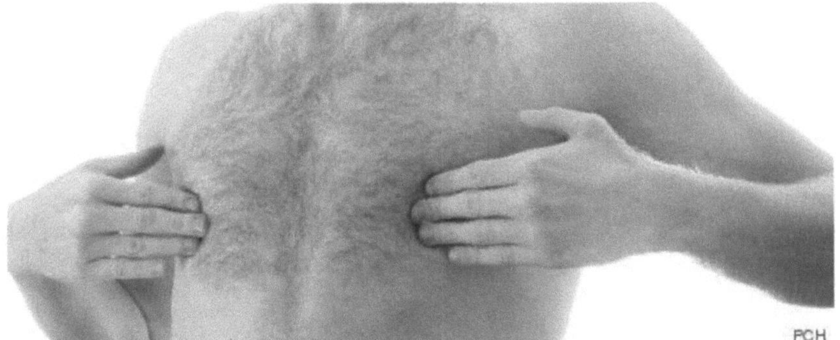

Figura 11: Male Breast Cancer

Source:<https://www.huffpostbrasil.com/2015/07/31/cancer-de-mama-masculino-tudo-que-voce-precisa-saber_a_21690843/>. Accessed on 09/08/2018.

SYMPTOMS OF MALE BREAST CANCER

Normally the symptoms of breast cancer are the same as in women, so men should carry out the same procedures to avoid the disease.

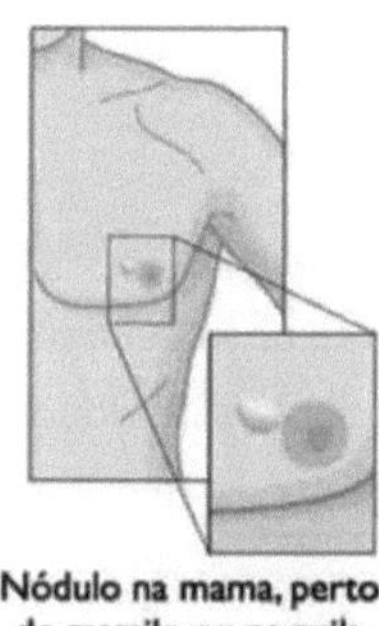

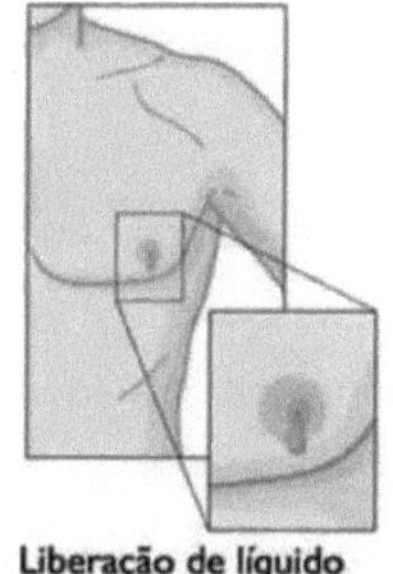

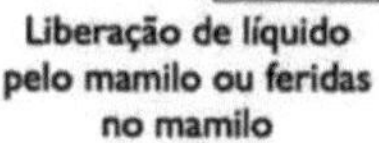

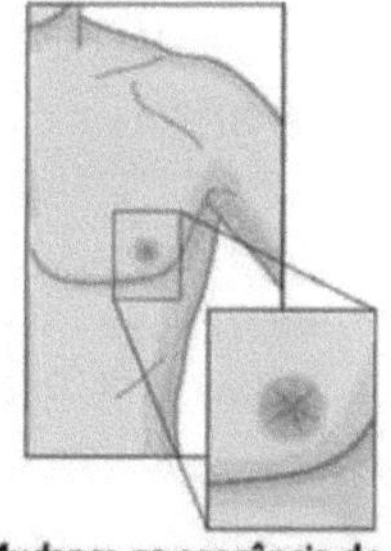

Figure 12: Symptoms of Male Breast Cancer

Source: <http://www.imeb.com.br/12-sintomas-do-cancer-de-mama/>. Accessed on: 09/08/2018.

HISTOLOGICAL TYPE OF BREAST CANCER

Within the histological profile of breast cancer there are several types, but there are some that are quite rare, or even a tumour may have combinations of types.

COMMON TYPES OF BREAST CANCER

- *Ductal Carcinoma In Situ:* One of the most common non-invasive cancers. Also called intraductal carcinoma, it affects the ducts of the breast, which are the channels that produce milk. This carcinoma doesn't invade other tissues, much less spread through the bloodstream. The membrane lining the tumour doesn't rupture, so the cancer cells are concentrated only in that nodule, but there can be several foci of these cells in a single breast. This type of carcinoma has the potential to become invasive (AMERICAN CANCER SOCIETY, 2017);
- *Lobular Carcinoma In Situ:* This carcinoma originates *in* the breast lobules, i.e. near the milk-producing glands. It is usually multifocal, i.e. it presents in several areas of the breast, but it does not have the capacity to reach other tissues (AMERICAN CANCER SOCIETY, 2017);
- *Invasive Ductal Carcinoma:* It can also be called infiltrating, it is very common when talking about invasive neoplasms, it starts in the milk duct, breaks the wall and grows in the adipose tissue of the breast and can even invade other tissues as the stage of the disease progresses, it invades other tissues through the lymphatic vessels and veins. It is characterised by the presence of one or more hormone receptors on cell surfaces (AMERICAN CANCER SOCIETY, 2017);
- *Invasive Lobular Carcinoma:* This carcinoma begins in the milk-producing glands, it can invade other tissues, growing and spreading to healthy tissues, in its structure it usually has estrogen and progesterone on the surface of the cells, it is

much more likely to affect both breasts (AMERICAN CANCER SOCIETY, 2017).

LESS COMMON TYPES OF BREAST CANCER

- *Inflammatory Carcinoma:* A rare type of carcinoma, known as triple negative. It is one of the most aggressive forms of breast cancer, it presents as an inflammation of the breast and takes on a large proportion, it also starts in the milk-producing glands, and has a high chance of advancing to other areas of the body, metastasising (AMERICAN CANCER SOCIETY, 2017).
- *Paget's disease:* This histological type affects the areola or the nipples, and can even affect both at the same time. It is a rare type, characterised by alterations to the skin of the nipple, causing crusts and even inflammation, but it can also be asymptomatic, showing no symptoms. Some scholars claim that Paget's disease begins in the breast ducts and progresses to the epidermis; other scholars claim that the cancer cells develop in the terminal portion of the ducts, where they join the epidermis (AMERICAN CANCER SOCIETY, 2017).
- *Phylloid tumour:* This is a very rare type of neoplasm that begins in the stroma (a connective tissue) of the breast and contrasts with carcinomas that develop in the ducts and lobules (AMERICAN CANCER SOCIETY, 2017).
- *Angiosarcoma:* In this neoplasm, the cells form in the blood vessels or lymphatics, and its incidence in the breast is extremely rare (AMERICAN CANCER SOCIETY, 2017).

SPECIAL TYPES OF INVASIVE BREAST CARCINOMA

The special types are subtypes of invasive neoplasms, in some cases they may have a better prognosis than the ductal and lobular invasive carcinomas themselves:

- *Adenoid cystic carcinoma: This* rare neoplasm has a slow biological course and normally does not metastasise to the axillary lymph nodes (Ritto *et al.,* 2005).
- *Mucinous carcinoma:* This is an uncommon histological type with a higher incidence in older women and slow growth. The tumour itself has an extremely soft consistency and a jelly-like appearance. The rate of patients who survive is usually higher than for other carcinomas, and metastases can occur in the lymph nodes in less than 20 per cent of cases (XAVIER, 2009).
- *Medullary* carcinoma*:* Known as basal carcinoma, it is a subgroup of cancer that is most often detected as "interval cancer". This subtype of carcinoma often has the morphological appearance of a benign lesion and since this histological type is

associated with high-risk patients, it is important to study these lesions and their imaging characteristics (MATHEUS *etaL,* 2008).

- Papillary carcinoma: This is a special histology that grows in a papillary shape inside cysts. It can be confused with carcinoma in situ, but its structure is papillary and has the appearance of malignant cancer cells (BARCELOS *etaL,* 1999).
- *Tubular carcinoma:* Among the special histological types, this is the most important, because this carcinoma has a good prognosis and low ability to metastasise (AMERICAN CANCER SOCIETY, 2017).

Other types can be much worse in terms of prognosis than invasive carcinoma itself. Such as:

- *Metaplastic carcinoma:* This can be confused with invasive ductal carcinoma, but it has some differences that help with diagnosis. It is a heterogeneous tumour that contains ductal carcinoma cells interspersed with fusiform areas, as well as squamous, chondroid or adenosquamous elements, which may be due to its myoepithelial origin (ABRAHÃO *et al.,* 2014 *apud* ESBAH *et al.,* 2012).
- Micropapillary carcinoma: This is an extremely rare variant of invasive carcinoma. It is formed by massive epithelial tumours with a micropapillary appearance without a fibrovascular axis being evident. This tumour is normally associated with lymphovascular tumour invasion and axillary metastasis with extracapsular extension (OLIVEIRA; SILVA, .
- *Mixed carcinoma:* This type is characterised by ductal and lobular carcinoma, a lesion that has malignant epithelial characteristics (in situ and invasive) in the breast ducts and lobules.

Although these subtypes exist, they are usually only treated as invasive ductal or lobular carcinomas.

RISK FACTORS

When it comes to risk factors, there are always various ways in which this pathology can develop.

FAMILY HISTORY

When it comes to family history, it is always heredity, that is, genetics. Within genetics, it is important to note the following points according to the *American Cancer Society* (2017):

- First-degree relatives who have had the condition;
- At least one first-degree relative and two second- or third-degree relatives;
- Two first-degree relatives, at least one who manifested it before the age of 45;
- A first-degree relative with bilateral breast cancer;
- A first-degree relative with the disease and one or more relatives with ovarian cancer;
- One second- or third-degree relative with breast cancer and two or more with ovarian cancer;
- Three or more second- or third-degree relatives with the disease;
- Two second- or third-degree relatives with breast cancer and one or more with ovarian cancer.

AGE

Women between the ages of 40 and 69 are the most affected, because they are exposed to the hormone estrogen. Around the age of 50, the chances start to decrease, but the possibility is not ruled out, the only thing that happens from that age onwards is that hormone levels start to have an upward curve *(AMERICAN CANCER SOCIETY, 2017).*

EARLY MENSTRUATION

Menstruation is a risk factor because with menarche, a young woman starts to produce more oestrogen hormones, and when there are high amounts in the body, this causes the body to proliferate breast cells in a disorderly fashion, making it easier for the tumour to develop. The earlier the menstruation, it's a sign that the ovaries have started to intensify their production of the hormone early on and it means that they'll have more time with oestrogen throughout their lives *(AMERICAN CANCER SOCIETY, 2017).*

LATE MENOPAUSE

As long as the menstrual cycle does not cease, the ovary continues to produce oestrogen, which contributes to making the mammary glands prone to cancer cell growth *(AMERICAN CANCER SOCIETY, 2017).*

HORMONE REPLACEMENT

When women are in the climacteric process, which is when they experience a set of symptoms due to hormonal variations, it is necessary to control hormones in order to reduce the symptoms of this process. This replacement mainly includes steroids such as oestrogen and progesterone, which increase the chances of cell proliferation *(AMERICAN CANCER SOCIETY, 2017).*

HIGH CHOLESTEROL

Cholesterol becomes high when there is an excess of fat in the body, and fat serves as a raw material for the production of oestrogen. As a result, women with high cholesterol have a higher production of this hormone, increasing their risk of breast cancer *(AMERICAN CANCER SOCIETY, 2017).*

OBESITY

When a person is overweight or obese, this is a major risk factor for developing the condition, especially during the menopause. This is due to the fact that excess adipose tissue is a new producer of hormones, due to the action of enzymes, the fat that is stored in the breast is converted into estrogen *(AMERICAN CANCER SOCIETY, 2017).*

NO PREGNANCY

When a woman becomes pregnant, her oestrogen load decreases and, consequently, when she breastfeeds, the same process occurs, simply because the action of the child feeding through the breast causes the mammary glands to be stimulated, thus decreasing the oestrogen in the bloodstream *(AMERICAN CANCER SOCIETY, 2017).*

RISK INJURIES

When the patient has any type of mutation in the breast, whether or not it is related to the neoplasm, it can lead to the formation of tumours *(American Cancer Society, 2017).* An example of this are the cells that make benign tumours. When they appear, prevention work should begin with the person, so that they don't become malignant and then lead to higher costs for everyone involved.

ANTERIOR BREAST TUMOUR

When an individual has already had a neoplasm in the breast, there can be an increased chance of a new tumour; this is known as recurrent cancer *(AMERICAN CANCER SOCIETY, 2017).*

BREAST CANCER INCIDENCE

Cancer is a pathology that has become a major public health problem worldwide. According to INCA, the number of new cancer cases in Brazil in 2011 was almost 500,000.

Primary localisation	Estimates of new cases		
	Male	Female	Total
Prostate	52.350	-	52.350
Female breast	-	49.240	49.240
Trachea, bronchi and lungs	17.800	9.830	27.630
Colon and rectum	13.310	14.800	28.110
Stomach	13.820	7.680	21.500

Cervix	-	18.430	18.430
Oral cavity	10.330	3.790	14.120
Oesophagus	7.890	2.740	10.630
Leukaemias	5.240	4.340	9.580
Melanoma skin	2.960	2.970	5.930
Other locations	59.130	78.770	137.900
Subtotal	182.830	192.590	375.420
Non-melanoma skin	53.410	60.440	113.850
All neoplasms	236.240	253.030	489.270

Source: INCA, 2009

Figura 13: Cancer estimates according to INCA

TAKEN FROM: BRAZIL, INCA. 2011.

According to a survey carried out in 2006, Rio de Janeiro - RJ was the Brazilian city with the most breast cancer cases, followed by Porto Alegre - RS (BRASIL, 2006).

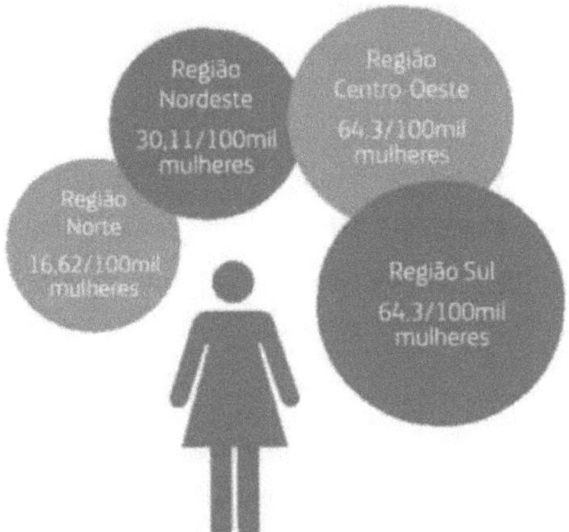

Figura 14: Breast Cancer by Region in 2014.

Source: <http://fundacaotelefonica.org.br/noticias/telefonica-vivo-contra-o-cancer-de-mama/>. Accessed on: 08/08/2018.

Breast neoplasms can appear in any of its structures: epidermis, mesenchyme and glandular epithelium. Breast carcinoma is found more often in the left breast than the right, and approximately 4% of cancers are bilateral or sequences in the same breast. Around 50 per cent arise in the

upper outer quadrant of the breast, 10 per cent in another quadrant (upper inner, lower outer and lower inner) and 20 per cent in the central region (XAVIER, 2009).

According to INCA (2018), in 2018 there will be 59,700 cases of breast cancer in Brazil alone, with a risk of 56.33 per 100,000 women. In 2012, there were an estimated 1.67 million new cases worldwide, which is equivalent to 25% of all cancer cases in the world (INCA, 2018).

Deaths totalled an estimated 522,000 in 2012 alone, representing a total of 14.7% of deaths worldwide. In underdeveloped countries, it is the second leading cause of death due to neoplasms, second only to lung cancer, while in developed countries it is the leading cause of death due to cancer. Among the mortality rates for overall female deaths in Brazil, it corresponds to a total of 3% (INCA, 2018).

CENÁRIO ATUAL
IMAMA
INCIDÊNCIA EM 100 MIL MULHERES:
90,20 Incidência no RS
56,20 Incidência No BR
130,99 Incidência em POA
No Mundo é o 2º mais frequente
53,90% casos avançados
1mm de aumento no nódulo, diminui em 1% a chance de cura
Detectado em fase inicial tem 95% de cura
Fonte: INCA

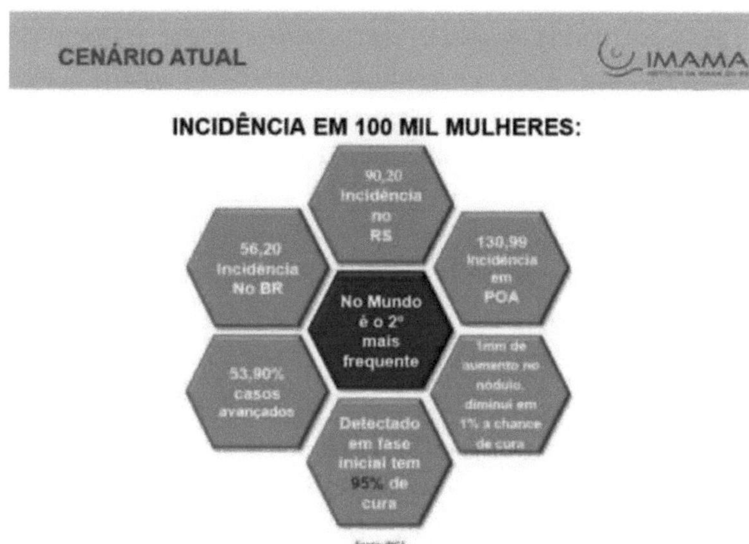

Figura 15: Breast Cancer Incidence

Source: < http://www.solidariedade.org.br/noticias/solidariedade-mulher-promove-acoes-do-outubro-rosa-no-rs/>. Accessed on: 08/08/2018.

There is a wide variation by region: in the South and Southeast of Brazil, 6.6 women die for every 100,000 women; in the North and Northeast, the figure rises by more than 100 per cent to 14 for every 100,000 women (INCA, 2018).

In order for this neoplasm to reduce its mortality rate, there needs to be early detection and adequate planning for screening. It is estimated that at least one in three cases of breast cancer can be cured.

According to RBA data (2018), in a report on breast cancer:

> *"Data from the Oncology Observatory shows the cost of treating early-stage breast cancer: R$11,373 per patient with pre-menopausal breast cancer and R$49,488 in post-menopausal cases. In the more advanced stages, these figures reach R$ 55,125 and R$ 93,241, respectively. And each female life lost to cancer causes an average loss of R$145,000 in the economy" (RBA, 2018).*

There is a low incidence of this neoplasm in men, but it can usually be diagnosed after the age of 60.

Around 56% of breast lesions do not have a specific histological type, they are only classified as invasive cancer (BRASIL, 2006).

Ductal in situ breast cancer is the most common of the non-invasive types, affecting between 94% and 98% of cases, while lobular in situ usually affects between 2% and 6% of the population with the neoplasm. As for invasive, the invasive ductal type affects around 65% to 85% of the population with this neoplasm. Paget's disease can affect between 0.5% and 4.3% of the population, making it a rare pathology. The medullary invasive subtype represents around 2% to 7%, occurring more frequently in younger patients. Tubular carcinoma affects around 2% and patients have a 90% chance of being cured (BRASIL, 2006; XAVIER, 2009).

The high incidence rate in 2018, with a total of 60,000 new cases this year alone, is a cause for great concern, because there is a lack of investment in so many areas of public health - investment in continuing education for prevention throughout the year, not just in one season.

PREVENTION

One of the main methods of diagnosing breast cancer at an early stage is mammography, which can detect non-palpable alterations and thus guarantee early treatment of the pathology, a less aggressive and more effective treatment, with better aesthetic results and significantly reduced adverse events. However, despite the fact that several studies have shown a reduction in breast cancer mortality through mass mammographic screening, its effectiveness is controversial, especially in women under 50. Despite this, mass mammography screening has been encouraged and carried out on women from the age of 40 and even with its limitations, it is still the best method for preventing breast cancer (Sclowitz *et al.,* 2005).

Breast cancer prevention is not entirely effective, due to the many factors associated with the disease and the fact that many of these factors are not modifiable. Prevention is therefore based on controlling risk factors and encouraging protective factors that are considered modifiable (Sclowitz *et al.,* 2005; INCA, 2008).

There are studies that say that through diet, nutrition and physical activity it is possible to reduce a woman's risk of developing breast cancer by up to 28 per cent (INCA, 2008).

PINK OCTOBER

Pink October is a movement that was created in the United States in the 1990s, when Susan G. Komen organised a race for the cure in New York City to encourage public participation in controlling and fighting breast cancer. The date is honoured annually with the aim of sharing information about the disease and raising awareness about the importance of early detection of the pathology (INCA, 2018).

The event starts on 1 October until 31 October and is a month of awareness, information and campaigning for this very important cause that affects many people in the country and around the world (INCA, 2018).

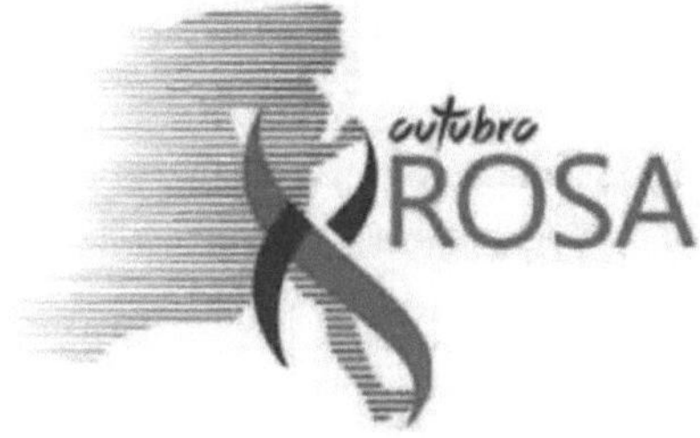

Figura 16: Pink October.

Source: <http://desabafosocial.com.br/blog/2016/10/31/outubro-das-mulheres/> Accessed on: 15/08/2018.

DIAGNOSIS

The diagnosis of this pathology can be made by a variety of means, including clinical examination, where the diagnosis is made by a doctor, or by imaging tests such as mammography, ultrasound or MRI, the last two of which are only used to complement the diagnosis made by mammography.

When the disease is discovered, tests are ordered to find out the stage of the disease, such as blood tests, chest x-rays, abdominal ultrasound and bone scintigraphy, as well as other more specific tests if necessary.

CHAPTER 3

BREAST SELF-EXAMINATION

Self-examination is a form of prevention for women, but it is often the first step towards diagnosing breast cancer. It is considered to be a preventative measure, because women should carry out this test at least once a month, three to five days after their menstrual period, because all the swelling from that period has gone and it won't interfere with feeling lumps.

It is recommended that any woman after the age of twenty who has a case of breast cancer in her family, or any woman over the age of forty, should carry out a breast self-examination in order to diagnose the disease before it reaches a more serious stage.

To carry out the self-examination, you need to stand in front of a mirror, either standing up or lying down, and follow these steps:

- 1º With dropped arms;
- 2º Raise your arms and look at your breasts;
- 3º It is recommended that you place your hands on the pelvic area, applying pressure to check for any changes in the breast surface.
- 4º Observe the size, shape, colour of the breasts, bumps, lumps, bumps, bumps.

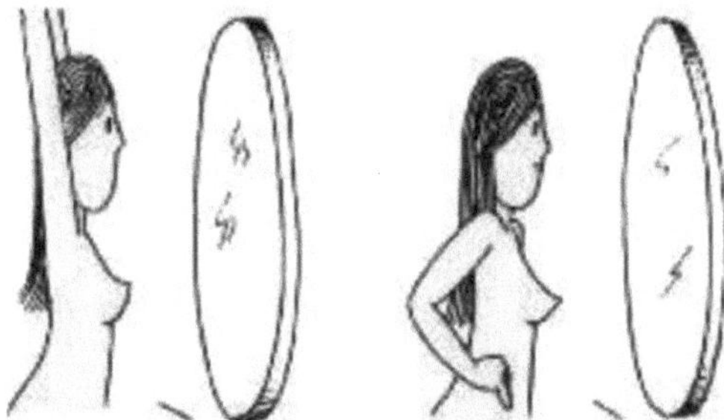

Figure 17: Mirror observation.

Source: < http://www.saudeemmovimento.com.br/conteudos/conteudo_exibe1 .asp?cod_noticia=1219>. Accessed on 07/08/2018.

After observing, palpation should be performed, if standing:

- 1º You should raise your left/right arm, placing your hand behind your head;
- 2º Palpate with the digital pulps carefully with the opposite hand from the side you are checking in circular movements, from bottom to top, so that you can check for lumps in the breast area. It is important to remember that the fingers of the hand should be together and straight, and after palpation you should press lightly on the nipples to check if any liquid/secretion is coming out of that nipple;

- 3° carry out the same steps on the other breast.

If the woman wishes to perform the self-exam lying down, she must follow these steps:

- 1° You should lie down and place your right/left arm on the back of your neck;

- 2° Place a cushion or towel under your right/left shoulder to make it more comfortable;

- 3° Palpate with the digital pulps carefully with the opposite hand from the side you are checking in circular movements, from bottom to top, so that you can check for lumps in the breast area. It is important to remember that the fingers of the hand should be together and straight, and after palpation you should press lightly on the nipples to check if any liquid/secretion is coming out of the nipple;

- 4° Repeat the same process on the breast that was not examined.

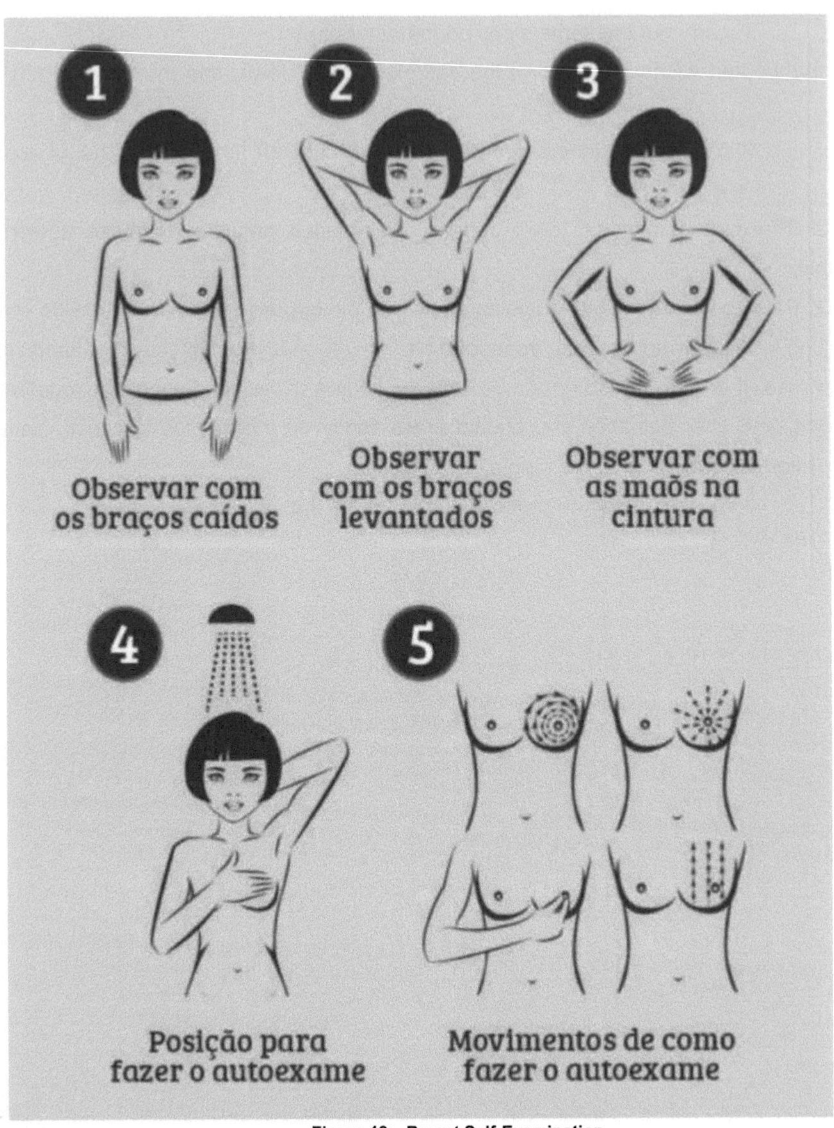

Figura 18: Breast Self-Examination.

Source: <http://www.uepb.edu.br/clinica-de-enfermagem-promove-orientacao-sobre-autoexame-para- prevencao-do-cancer-de-mama/>. Accessed on 07/08/2018.

MAMMOGRAPHY

Mammography is the standard test for early detection of breast cancer, it is important for all women, it can visualise around 90% of breast cancers.

cases, before the tumour has a more serious stage (NASCIMENTO; PITTA, RÊGO, 2015).

The aim of this examination is to reproduce detailed images with high spatial resolution of the internal structure of the breast in order to identify changes in the breast (NASCIMENTO; PITTA, RÊGO, 2015).

INCA (2018) recommends that women undergo screening at least once every two years from the age of 50. The Brazilian Society of Mastology, on the other hand, recommends that it be done once a year, from the age of 40, in order to carry out effective screening.

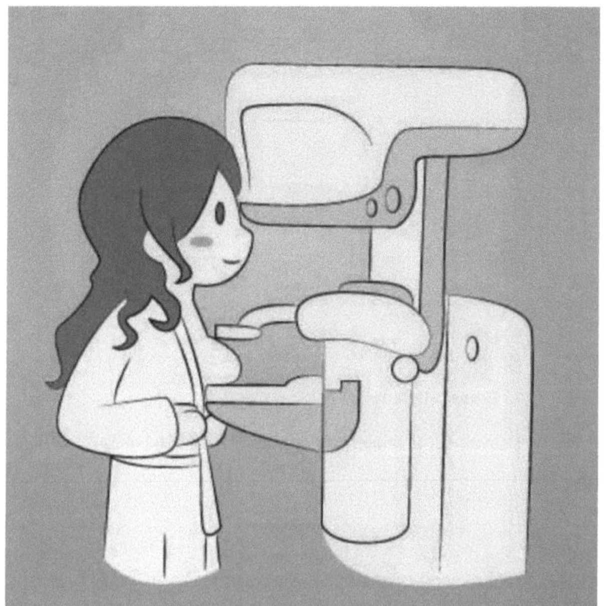

Figura 19: Breast Self-Examination.

Source: <http://www.uopeccan.org.br/noticias/uopeccan-vai-as-ruas-para-agendar-mammograms/attachment/mannography/>. Accessed on 09/08/2018.

Mammography is carried out using equipment called a mammography machine (just like X-ray equipment), which compresses the breast so that it offers high-quality images to make an optimum diagnosis. The breast needs to be compressed in order for the examination to be carried out effectively, however uncomfortable the pain may be (NASCIMENTO; PITTA, RÊGO, 2015).

BREAST ULTRASOUND

Breast ultrasound is a complement to mammography and it is thanks to this procedure that we are able to differentiate between a cyst and a nodule in the breast region (INCA, 2018).

The advantages of this form of diagnosis are that it is not an invasive procedure, is well tolerated by patients, and provides extra information to improve the physical examination and mammography. For patients who have dense breasts, the mammogram would ignore some alterations, but the ultrasound would be unbearable (NASCIMENTO; PITTA, RÊGO, 2015).

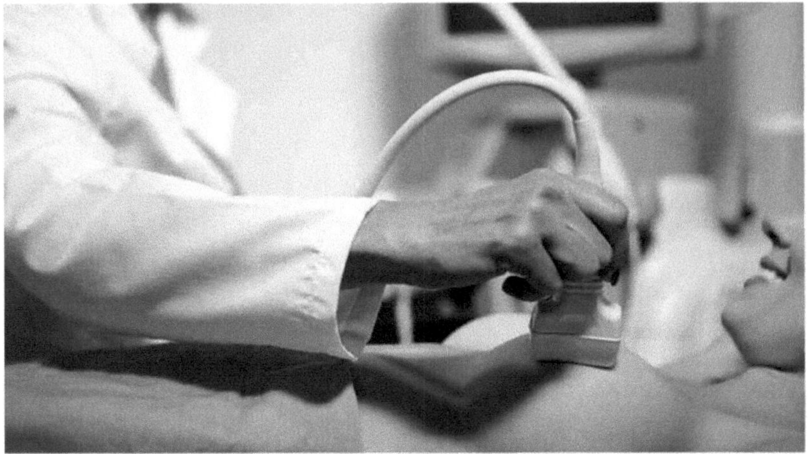

Figura 20: Breast ultrasound.

Source: <https://www.magicmaman.com/, tout-savoir-sur-l-echographie-mammaire,3422864.asp>. Accessed on 07/08/2018.

BREAST MRI

This procedure is indicated for screening women at high risk, women with a family history or suspicion, and even women who have already had cancer once and are suspected of having it again. MRI is also indicated when it has not been detected by mammography or ultrasound (AMERICAN CANCER SOCIETY, 2016).

Studies show that magnetic resonance imaging is more effective in the differential diagnosis between benign and malignant lesions, due to the fact that this form of diagnosis demonstrates the morphological characteristics of the tumour in greater detail (NASCIMENTO; PITTA, RÊGO, 2015).

This procedure has more advantages over mammography and ultrasound, such as: less exposure to radiation, better visualisation, location and morphology of malignant lesions and the real extent of the cancer, and we can carry out less aggressive treatment. The disadvantages are that it is difficult to identify whether it is a malignant or benign lesion, it has a high cost and can increase the number of surgeries and biopsies without there being any bearable needs (NASCIMENTO; PITTA, RÊGO, 2015).

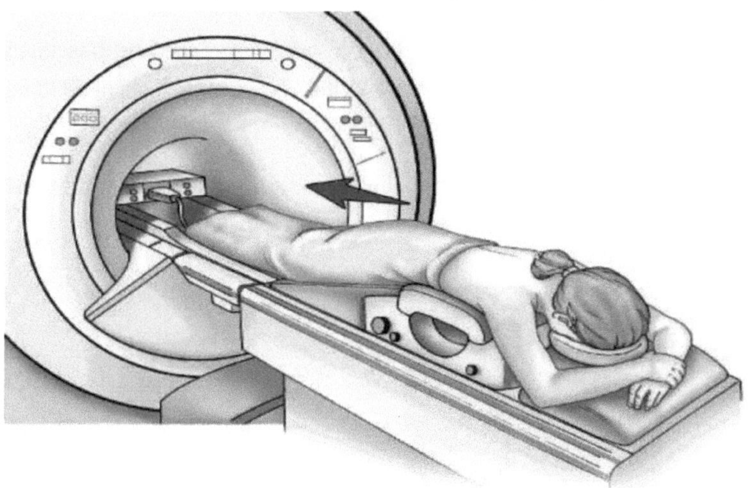

Figura 21: Breast MRI.

Source: < http://www.oncoguia.org.br/conteudo/ressonancia-magnetica-das-mamas/10876/264/ >. Accessed on 07/08/2018.

BI-RADS

It is a classification used to classify whether or not there are nodules in the breast region, and it promotes standardisation in reports (VIEIRA; TOIGO, 2002). BIRADS is the abbreviation *for "Breast Imaging Reporting and Data System".* This standardisation is used to estimate the chance of an image being cancerous or not (VIEIRA; TOIGO, 2002).

Its main objective is to avoid confusion in mammography reports. It does not estimate the degree of growth or the type of tumour, but it does indicate the chances in percentages of an individual having cancer. Normally there are some cysts, nodules or calcifications, but these are benign and there is no chance of cancer in the future (VIEIRA; TOIGO, 2002).BIRADS has a category from 0 to 6, in each category there is a percentage for cancer and the behaviour that the doctor should take in each situation:

TABLE 2: BIRADS classification.

BIRADS	SIGNIFICANCE	PORCETAGE	MEDICAL CONDUCT
0	It wasn't possible to assess the breast properly.	It is not possible to estimate.	Carry out additional tests.
1	Normal.	Very low.	Annual control.
2	Benign changes.	Very low.	Annual control.
3	Probably benign.	2%	Follow up with a mammogram every six months.
4A	Low risk.	20%	Needs to be assessed by biopsy
4B	Moderate risk.	20%	Needs to be assessed by biopsy
4C	High Cancer Risk.	20%	Needs to be assessed by biopsy
5	High Cancer Risk.	95%	Perform a biopsy.

6	Presence of malignant cells	100%	Oncological treatment.

- BIRADS 0: This classification is an unknown, it means that something has been detected, but it can't define the degree of what is in the breast, other tests need to be carried out to define it.
- BIRADS 1 and 2: This is considered normal, but it may evolve to 3 or 4 as you get older, but it is associated with benign and malignant breast diseases.

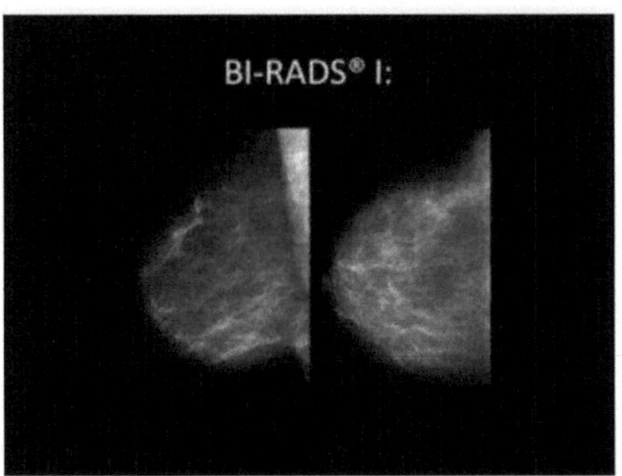

Figura 22: BI-RADS I

Source: <https://www.einstein.br/noticias/noticia/o-que-e-birads>. Accessed on 08/08/2018.

-BIRADS 3: This type requires six-monthly screening for 1 or 2 years. If there are no changes, it can be classified as BIRADS 2. Within this classification, as the risk is very low, there is no need for a biopsy.

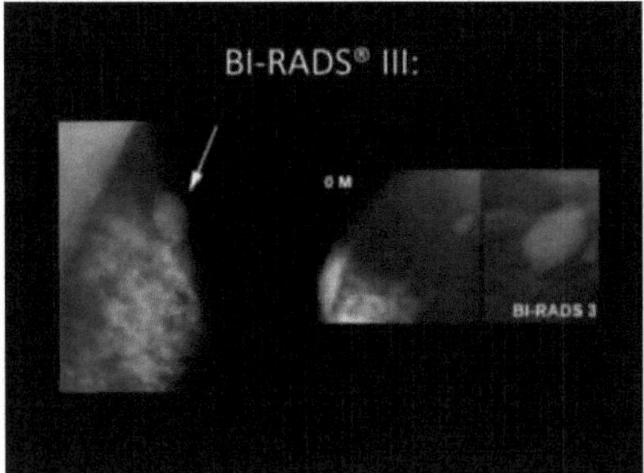

Figure 23: BI-RADS Iii

Source: <https://www.einstein.br/noticias/noticia/o-que-e-birads>. Accessed on 08/08/2018.

BI-RADS 4: When this classification is presented, a biopsy is required. It can be done with a fine or coarse needle. Depending on the biopsy, there may be a number of reports, such as: Benign (annual check-up only, returning to BI-RADS 2); Suspicious (there is an alteration, but the material needs to be removed for a reliable diagnosis); Malignant (oncological treatment required).

-BIRADS 5: The risk is extremely high, surgery is compulsory, a biopsy must be carried out before surgery, but the nodule must be completely removed .

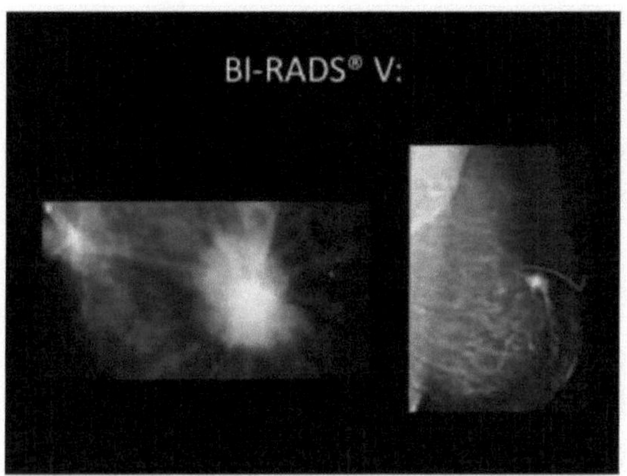

Figure 24: BI-RADS V

Source: <https://www.einstein.br/noticias/noticia/o-que-e-birads>. Accessed on 08/08/2018

- BIRADS 6: This case requires oncological, surgical and other types of follow-up to treat the neoplasm.

BIOPSY

A biopsy is the removal of a small amount of tissue for anatomical and pathological assessment of whether or not cancer is present. The sample that is removed during the biopsy is examined and analysed by a pathologist, a doctor who specialises in interpreting laboratory tests and evaluating cells, tissues and organs in order to diagnose pathology. If there are cancerous cells, the pathologist determines the corresponding type of breast cancer (AMERICAN CANCER SOCIETY, 2017).

There are various types of biopsy. The main types used to diagnose breast cancer are as follows:

- *Fine Needle Aspiration Puncture (FNAP):* Removal of a cellular sample from suspicious breast tissue for examination. A 20/21G needle coupled to a syringe is used for the procedure to aspirate the tissue. The positioning of this needle is guided by ultrasound (AMERICAN CANCER SOCIETY, 2017).

- *Core biopsy:* this is the removal of tissue fragments with a slightly thicker calibre needle than the FNAB, attached to a special gun. Positioning of the biopsy needle can be guided by stereotactic digital mammography or ultrasound. The procedure is performed under local anaesthesia (AMERICAN CANCER SOCIETY, 2017).
- *Surgical biopsy:* this is done in the operating theatre during surgery and has a great advantage because the margins are safer (AMERICAN CANCER SOCIETY, 2017).
- *Lymph node biopsy:* it is observed whether the lymph nodes are altered, now if not the axillary nodes are investigated for metastases (AMERICAN CANCER SOCIETY, 2017).

TREATMENT

When we talk about breast cancer treatment, we have to consider the major differences that occur in a woman's life during this process, because it can change her appearance a great deal, leading to major problems of acceptance.

This stage of cancer should be carried out by a multidisciplinary team, as the woman will need a variety of healthcare services (BARROS; BARBOS; GEBRIM*, et al.,* 2001).

CHEMIOTHERAPY

This treatment uses drugs to destroy the cancer, which can be administered intravenously or orally. Chemotherapy is administered into the bloodstream in order to target cancer cells throughout the body (AMERICAN CANCER SOCIETY, 2016).

According to the American Cancer Society (2016) there are several types of treatment:

- Adjuvant chemotherapy: This is given after surgery to destroy cancer cells left over from the surgical procedure or even spread by imaging tests. This type of chemotherapy can reduce the risk of recurrence.
- Neoadjuvant chemotherapy: This is given before surgery to try to reduce the size of the tumour so that it can be removed during surgery. It is used more for advanced cancers. If the tumour doesn't shrink, the doctor will know how to deal with it and will change the drugs to be used for treatment.
- Chemotherapy for metastatic disease: This is used as the main treatment for the disease.

Chemotherapy usually has some side effects, these are: hair loss; nail changes; mouth sores; loss or increase in appetite; nausea and vomiting; diarrhoea; infection (due to the immune system); bruising or bleeding (due to a decrease in platelets); fatigue (due to a decrease in red blood cells). These effects disappear quickly after the end of the chemotherapy section, some symptoms can be reduced through medication, but other effects can appear during the medication process, among them are (AMERICAN CANCER SOCIETY, 2016):

- Neuropathy: Some of the drugs used in this type of treatment damage the nerves in the brain and spinal cord, causing symptoms such as tingling, sensitivity to cold or heat and weakness, especially in the hands and feet. Once the treatment is finished, these symptoms usually disappear. Among the drugs responsible for this effect are - Taxanes; Platinum agents; Vinorelbine; Erubulia and Ixabepilone (AMERICAN CANCER SOCIETY, 2016).
- Hand-Foot Syndrome: Causes irritation of the palms of the hands and soles of the feet. Symptoms include numbness, tingling and redness. In worse cases it can cause oedema, bringing discomfort and in some cases pain. The drugs that can cause this effect are Capecitabine and Doxorubicin (AMERICAN CANCER SOCIETY, 2016).
- Chemo Brain or Chemotherapy Fog: Some women may have problems with concentration and memory, which can last for a long time. However, it is something that happens over a number of years, even when treatment has finished (AMERICAN CANCER SOCIETY, 2016).
- Fatigue: This is an effect that can occur over a number of years. It can be controlled, when symptoms appear the doctor should be assessed, and so the doctor will prescribe something to improve fatigue (AMERICAN CANCER SOCIETY, 2016).
- Heart Problems: This can be referred to as cardiomyopathy. The drug that causes the problem - doxorubicin, epirubicin and some other drugs can cause more of these problems (AMERICAN CANCER SOCIETY, 2016).
- Menstrual Changes and Fertility Problems: Young women experience a delay in the menstrual cycle. During early menopause and infertility can occur and may be permanent. For women with hormone receptor-positive breast cancer, some types of hormonal birth control are not a good option (AMERICAN CANCER SOCIETY, 2016).
- Risk of Leukaemia: Due to the lowering of the immune system, some drugs can cause diseases such as myelodysplastic syndrome or acute myeloid leukaemia (AMERICAN CANCER SOCIETY, 2016).

In both adjuvant and neoadjuvant treatment, chemotherapy is most effective with combinations of certain drugs. Many combinations are in use, but none is certain which is best.

The most common drugs used for adjuvant and neoadjuvant chemotherapy include:

- Anthracyclines - Doxorubicin and epirubicin;
- Taxanes - Paclitaxel and Docetaxel;
- 5-fluorouracil;
- Cyclophosphamide;
- Carboplatin.

When breast cancer is at an advanced stage, the drugs for this case are:

- Docetaxel;
- Paclitaxel;
- Platinum agents (cisplatin carboplatin);
- Vinorelbine;
- Capecitabine;
- Doxorubicin;
- Gemcitabine;
- Mitoxantrone;
- Ixabepilone;
- Eribulin.

Usually drugs such as carboplatin or cisplatin, together with gemcitabine, are used to treat advanced breast cancer.

HOMONIOTHERAPY

Within the human body there are glands that produce various types of hormones that cause cells to grow. With this, oestrogen, which helps female development, controls controlled and organised growth, but when there is disordered growth, cancer appears (INCA, 2018).

Hormone therapy is only used in breast cancer for cells that are positive for hormone receptors. Hormone therapy is a treatment carried out with estrogen and progesterone inhibitors, which prevents these hormones from reaching the breast cells so that tumour cells don't multiply.

The main drugs used in hormone treatment are:

- Tamoxifen: This drug blocks passage via hormone receptors located on cancer cells, so the hormone does not penetrate the cell and does not cause growth (INCA, 2018).
- Aromatosis inhibitors: This drug blocks the enzyme responsible for converting adrenal

hormones into female hormones, which is located in adipose tissue (INCA, 2018).

- Fulvestrant: This drug reduces the amount of cellular hormone receptors (INCA, 2018).

This therapy reduces the risk of breast cancer returning; it prevents tumour cells from increasing in volume; it reduces the volume of masses; it reduces the chances of cancer in women with a genetic risk of the pathology (INCA, 2018).

Side effects are symptoms similar to those found during the climacteric process, i.e. hot flushes, night sweats, vaginal dryness, mood swings. Vaginal bleeding and deep vein thrombosis (these are rare effects). Altralgias, osteopenia or osteoporosis, due to which patients use aromatase inhibitors, loss of bone and/or muscle mass (INCA, 2018).

This treatment is usually well accepted by all those who use it, which is why it is one of the most widely used (INCA, 2018).

TRANSTUZAMA ADJUVANT (ANTIBODY)

This therapy was a new drug that was used to treat cancer, initially it was used in cases of advanced stages that had already metastasised and today it is used in the early stages.

In this therapy, a humanised monoclonal antibody acts on the extracellular site of the receptor for human epidermal growth factor. It is approved for patients with invasive breast cancer. Under normal conditions, these receptors regulate cell growth, proliferation and survival.

It adds to adjuvant chemotherapy in both disease survival and overall survival, and is the only monoclonal antibody to produce success when used as an adjuvant therapy. The duration for this treatment is from nine weeks to two years.

RADIOTHERAPY

It is the type of treatment that uses ionising radiation to destroy or inhibit the growth of cancer cells. There are numerous types of radiation, but the most commonly used are electromagnetic (x-rays or gamma rays) and electrons (AMERICAN CANCER SOCIETY, 2016).

According to the American Cancer Society (2016) and Barros, Barbos, Gebrim, ***et al*** (2001) most women are not indicated for this type of treatment, but some situations should be taken into account, such as:

- After conservative surgery, to reduce the chance of recurrence in the breast or nearby lymph nodes;

- After mastectomy, especially if the tumour is more than 5 cm in diameter;
- If the patient had already metastasised.

There are two types of radiotherapy for breast cancer:

- External radiotherapy:

This is the most common type of treatment for breast cancer. It consists of irradiating the treatment in fractional doses, the patient feels nothing during the application, which lasts a few minutes a day. It is administered five times a week for around five or six weeks, but there are new treatments that increase the doses and reduce the number of sessions, in other words, reducing the duration of treatment (AMERICAN CANCER SOCIETY, 2016).

Within this treatment it is possible to have short-term side effects such as breast swelling, skin changes due to radiation and fatigue. These changes can be mild redness or even blistering and peeling, which can last a few months (AMERICAN CANCER SOCIETY, 2016).

There may be late side effects, such as: some women feel that the breast decreases in size and becomes firmer, there may be complications if the woman wishes to have breast reconstruction, there may be problems with breastfeeding, there may be algia in the shoulder region and the arm and hand, weakening of the ribs leading to fractures (AMERICAN CANCER SOCIETY, 2016).

When this procedure is performed, the type of surgery should be assessed, whether it was a mastectomy or breast-conserving surgery, and whether or not the lymph nodes were compromised (AMERICAN CANCER SOCIETY, 2016). After breast-conserving surgery, this procedure should be carried out regardless of histological type, age, use of chemotherapy or homonotherapy (BARROS; BARBOS; GEBRIM *et al.,* 2001). Post-mastectomy, on the other hand, is very controversial, according to Barros, Barbos, Gebrim *et al.* (2001), who say that it is the most appropriate procedure to avoid metastasis or a return of the pathology.

There are different types of treatment:

- ❖ Hypofractionated radiotherapy: The treatment is done in high doses for three weeks, it is for women who have had conservative breast surgery and without disease in the axillary lymph nodes, it can reduce side effects in the short term.
- ❖ Intraoperative radiotherapy: This type involves a single dose of radiation and is administered in the operating theatre once breast-conserving

surgery has been completed.

- ❖ 3D conformal radiotherapy: This type of radiotherapy is administered with special equipment, targeted at the area of the tumour. This allows the healthy breast to be spared. The treatment is carried out twice a day, five times a week, and is considered accelerated partial breast irradiation therapy.

- Internal radiotherapy or brachytherapy:

This therapy is carried out by inserting the radioactive material into or near the site that needs treatment, and it is possible that there may be some side effects inside, among which are: redness, bruising, breast pain, infection, injury to the fatty tissue area of the breast and rib fractures in rare cases (AMERICAN CANCER SOCIETY, 2016).

According to the American Cancer Society (2016) there are different types of treatment:

- ❖ Interstitial Brachytherapy: Several catheters with radioactive material are placed around the area of the breast where the tumour has been removed and left for a few days to release the necessary amount of dose for treatment, but this method is no longer used.
- ❖ Intracavitary Brachytherapy: This is the most common type of treatment. Different types of devices can be used, including MammoSite, SAVI, Axxent and Contura. Treatment is usually administered twice a day, for a total of five days.

CHAPTER 4

SURGERY

- *LUMPECTOMY*

According to the dictionary, it is a surgical procedure that removes only the breast lump and an adjacent margin of normal tissue. It can be used to diagnose breast cancer and for biopsy in the treatment of early-stage cancer (INCA, 2018).

- *QUADRANTECTOMY*

It is also called a tumorectomy, a partial mastectomy or segmental mastectomy, which consists of removing the segment or sector of the breast that has a tumour, the aim is to remove the tumour, the definition of how much of the breast is removed varies according to size and location (INCA, 2018).

- *MASTECTOMY*

Mastectomy is the total or partial removal of the breast, which may or may not be associated with the removal of the lymph nodes in the armpit. Speaking a little about the post-operative period of this surgery, the person needs to take certain precautions, mainly with the arm and movement on the same side as the operated breast (INCA, 2018).

It's important to know and take care that the operated site and the other breast should be examined monthly because the disease may return or something abnormal may be happening in the operated site, so taking care to observe changes in temperature or skin colour and the appearance of lumps should be reported to the doctor as soon as possible (INCA, 2018).

In the case of a bruise on the arm on the side where the breast was operated on, the patient should dress it every day and keep the wound protected until it heals completely. If the bruise doesn't improve and persists, don't hesitate and go to the doctor (INCA, 2018).

Once the surgical wound has completely healed, the skin should always be well moisturised with creams. It is recommended that if the patient is going to use external prostheses, they should only be fitted when the healing of the mastectomised area is complete and under medical supervision (INCA, 2018).

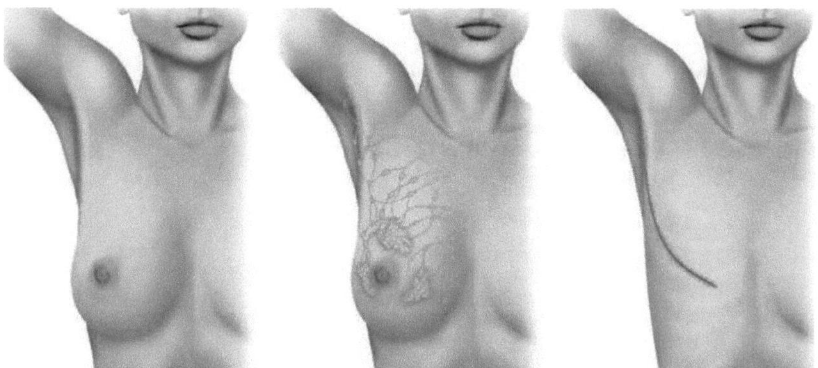

Figure 25: Mastectomy

Source: < http://dicionariosaude.com/mastectonnia/>. Accessed on 09/08/2018.

RESULTS FOR CREATING THEMES:

TABLE 3: Articles for creating themes

Title	Author(s)	Year of publication	Language / Country
The impact of mastectomy on women's lives.	ALMEIDA, RA.	2006	Portuguese / Brazil
Breast cancer: from discovery to recurrence	PINHO, LS; CAMPOS, ACS; FERNANDES, AFC; LOBO, SA.	2007	Portuguese / Brazil
The information needs of mastectomised women subsidising nursing care.	BARRETO, RAS; SUZUKI, K; LIMA, MA; MOREIRA, AA.	2008	Portuguese / Brazil
Physiotherapy in the rehabilitation of women operated on for breast cancer.	JAMMAL, ML; MACHADO, ARM; RODRIGUES, LR.	2008	Portuguese/Brazilian
Experiences and discourses of mastectomised women: negotiations and challenges of breast cancer.	COMIN, FS; SANTOS , MA; SOUZA, LV.	2009	Portuguese / Brazil
Stra tegies coping with breast cancer: a case study with families of mastectomised women.	TAVARES, JSC; TRAD, LAB.	2010	Portuguese / Brazil
The feelings of women after mastectomised.	MOURA, FMJSP; SILVA, MG; OLIVEIRA, SC; MOURA, LJSP.	2010	Portuguese / Brazil
Quality of life in women who have undergone mastectomy compared to those who have undergone conservative surgery: a literature review.	MAJEWSKI, JM; LOPES, ADF; DAVOGLIO, T; LEITE, JCC	2012	Portuguese / Brazil
Women with breast cancer: expressions of the social question during neoadjuvant chemotherapy treatment.	FRAZÃO, A; SKABA, MMFV.	2013	Portuguese/Brazilian
Legal rights of people with cancer: knowledge of users of a public oncology service	ROSA, LFA; GIRARDON-PERLINI, NMO; STAMM, B; COUTO, MS; CARDOSO, AL; BIRK, NM.	2014	Portuguese/Brazilian

Psychosocial adjustment after mastectomy - a look at quality of life.	FARIA, NC; FANGEL, LMV; ALMEIDA, AM; PRADO, MAS; CARLO, MMRP.	2016	Portuguese / Brazil
Breast cancer and emotional reactions: a review systematic.	ARAB, C; DEMONICO, BB; CORRE IA, CK; VILARINO, GT; ANDRADE, A.	2016	Portuguese / Brazil
Prophylactic surgery in hereditary breast cancer syndrome.	VIAL, IL; FUENZALIDA RR; PIZARRO, FC; ROJAS, VO; VIAL, GL.	2016	Spanish / Chile
Sitting time, body image and quality of life in women after breast cancer surgery.	BOING, L; ARAÚJO, CCR; PEREIRA, GS; MORATELLI, J; BENNETI, M; BORGATTO, AF; BERGAMANN, A; GUIMARÃES, ACA.	2017	Portuguese / Brazil
The meanings of breast cancer for women in the context of chemotherapy treatment.	MACHADO, MX; SOARES, DA; OLIVEIRA, SB.	2017	Portuguese / Brazil
Quality of life of mastectomised women enrolled in a rehabilitation programme.	GALDINO, AR; PEREIRA, LD; COSTA NETO, SB; BRANDÃO, CS; AMORIM, MHC.	2017	Portuguese / Brazil
Im portance of psychological support for mastectomised women: a review article.	RODRIGUES, NS; ORSINI, MRCA; MACHADO, AA; MONTIEL, JM; BARTHOLOMEU, D; TERTULIANO, IW.	2017	Portuguese / Brazil

The results of the related studies constituted five themes that identified the meaning of breast cancer treatment and mastectomy in women's lives. The themes identified were: Body image and sex life; Quality of life after mastectomy; Assistance and care for patients; Family context during the breast cancer process; Social and psychological context of breast cancer; Rights of breast cancer patients.

THEME: BODY IMAGE AND SEX LIFE AFTER BREAST CANCER

When it comes to body image, it means how a woman sees herself during and after breast cancer treatment and how this can affect her personal life (MOURA *et a!,* 2010).

Many women, when they discover they have breast cancer, start thinking that their image, their beauty, will be altered in one way or another (ALMEIDA, 2006).

The fear generated by the physical and emotional realisation that something will be missing from her body creates uncertainty as to whether she can continue to be a complete woman, simply because women portray their feminine essence through their hair, breasts and uterus, which are synonymous with the fact that a woman is complete (BARRETO *etal.,* 2008; MACHADO; SOARES; OLIVEIRA, 2017). The fact that breast cancer affects two extremely important parts of a woman totally affects her psychosocial and emotional factors (COMIN; SANTOS; SOUZA, 2009).

When she loses her hair during chemotherapy treatment, it is already an extremely delicate moment, because she can no longer see herself as whole (TAVARES; TRAD, 2010). From this moment on, the woman starts to have problems with her image, because she doesn't feel safe wearing the same clothes, doing the same make-up, going out in public places, because everyone will look at her with a feeling of pity.

Due to the feeling of fear of being belittled or being a *"laughing stock"* for not having any more hair, or using wigs, among other accessories, some women end up adhering to them (GALDINO *et a!,* 2017).

The most difficult moment for body image in cancer treatment is when the news comes through that a mastectomy will have to be performed (of any type). This is one of the most delicate moments in breast cancer treatment due to the fact that from this point onwards the woman will be completely mutilated, sometimes the advances that had already been made in how the patient was seeing herself completely recede, this procedure is something that will leave her without a part of the concept that many women have of what it is to be sensual and to be a woman (RODRIGUES *et al.,* 2017).

When the breast is removed, the woman no longer wants to look at herself in the mirror, she no longer feels desired and loved by her partner, she is ashamed to show her body to anyone, leading to various problems for the patient's self-image (ARAB *et a!,* 2016).

Due to the shame of their mutilated bodies, the traumas they carry, the lack of self-confidence, the pain, many end up losing interest in sex, start finding ways for their partner not to want them, not to touch them, damaging their marital relationship and in some cases even leading to divorce (ARAB *et aL,* 2016).

THEME: QUALITY OF LIFE AFTER MASTECTOMY

Quality of life is an individual's perception of their position in life in the context of the culture and value systems in which they live and in relation to their goals, expectations, standards and concerns (MAJEWSKI *et aL, 2011).* Quality of life can be assessed from the patient's point of view, referring to patients' appreciation and satisfaction with their functional level, compared to what they perceive to be possible or ideal (MAJEWSKI *et aL, 2011;* FARIA *et aL,* 2016/

In women with breast cancer it can be influenced by the type of surgery, the longer the surgery, the greater the difficulties in upper limb functionality, and the greater the morbidity, the more damage to general health, physical, functional, cognitive and social functions (BOING *et aL*, 2017; TAVARES; TRAD, 2010).

Mastectomy surgery often results in physical limitations in the collateral arm of women with breast cancer, with changes in their daily lives and deficits in autonomy (VIAL *etaL*, 2016).

When patients need to distance themselves from their professional occupation, this causes a feeling of decline in their productive capacity and discomfort caused by the idea of burdening family and friends. Accepting the change in the role of carer is an arduous task, mainly because they cannot perform all the functions they did before they fell ill (VIAL *etaL*, 2016; GALDINO *etaL*, 2017).

THEME: PATIENT CARE AND ASSISTANCE

All the studies selected addressed the issue of assistance and care. Each woman reacts in a different way to the pathology, but most women, from the moment they discover the illness, until the treatment and possible cure, improve their defence mechanisms such as: denial, rejection, anger, depression, distress and fear, until they reach the acceptance phase and seek a cure for the disease (BARRETO *et aL*, 2008; ARAB *et aL*, 2016; FARIA *et aL*, 2016).

The first thing to bear in mind throughout the process is that this assistance must be carried out in a comprehensive manner, i.e. with multi-professional support, with the support of family and friends, and especially the support of the patient (BARRETO *et al.,* 2008; MAJEWSKI *et al., 2011;* FARIA *et al.*, 2016; BOING *et al.*, 2017; GALDINO *et al.,* 2017/

Multiprofessional support has to take a holistic view of the client's life, since everyone around her is experiencing this moment together, so assistance and support should be for everyone, especially psychological support. The patient must focus on the moment of bodily changes, as depression can develop, so it is the role of the health team to identify this as soon as possible, in order to refer her to a psychologist, thus avoiding major consequences for this woman's life (BARRETO *et al.,* 2008; COMIN; SANTOS; SOUZA, 2009; TAVARES; TRAD, 2010).

Physiotherapy care, both pre and post-operatively, improves women's quality of life by preventing complications and promoting functional recovery. Normally, women who have undergone mastectomy are instructed in all their exercises and the sooner they start exercising after surgery, the easier their recovery will be (JAMMAL; MACHADO; RODRIGUES, 2008).

The family will be affected, as they will have to change their entire routine to focus on caring for their loved one with the illness (TAVARES; TRAD, 2010). Nurses and community health workers must carry out interventions because a simple conflict can become something huge and difficult to resolve.

Changes in people's daily lives can promote a state of equilibrium or imbalance, depending on people's comprehension or understanding of the situation, as well as the available means or devices of help and assistance used by those involved (RODRIGUES *etaL,* 2017).

It is also important to emphasise that Brazilian Law 9.797 of 1999 states that women who have undergone total or partial mastectomy are entitled to reconstructive plastic surgery, and in the event of technical and medical conditions, the procedure can take place immediately after the cancer has been removed (BARRETO *etaL*, 2008; GALDINO *etaL*, 2017;' RODRIGUES *etaL*, 2017).

If this doesn't happen at the time of removal, after recovering from surgery she will undergo a breast reconstruction procedure. Currently, there are numerous projects where micro-pigmentation tattoos are carried out, drawing the breast alveolus (RODRIGUES *et al.*, 2017).

The role of the care professional is to show that no matter how delicate a time the patient is going through, everything can be resolved if she has the strength and, above all, the will to fight for her life (BARRETO *et al.*, 2008; MAJEWSKI *et al., 2011).*

THEME: FAMILY CONTEXT DURING THE BREAST CANCER PROCESS

Within a family unit, women are always the protagonists, both in the eyes of family members and in the eyes of public policies, because women are seen as the carers, the people who manage to keep the house together even if they work outside, who manage to be the centre of everyone in the home, and when something happens to them, the family begins to be destabilised.

However many women are coping with breast cancer, the most difficult part during the whole process is the family, because at the same time as the woman doesn't want to tell the family that she's scared or has bigger problems, she can't show them in front of the patient for fear that her physical and mental state will worsen, and that the biggest fear is losing her loved one to a disease.

For women with breast cancer, according to Frazão and Skaba (2013), care for family members and especially children tends to be greater, so that in the future if something happens this family member doesn't feel abandoned by the woman while she is going through the pathological process. In some cases, women prefer the family to stay away, and always prioritise the children, because they want to spare them from suffering.

However, what can be a time of suffering for the family member can improve their treatment, because the support that the family brings to the patient gives them strength and encouragement to face the pathology with great vigour.

The more family support a woman has during treatment contributes to each stage of acceptance of the disease process, brings comfort, as well as awakening the courage to fight in search of a cure (PINHO *etal.,* 2007).

THEME: SOCIAL AND PSYCHOLOGICAL CONTEXT OF BREAST CANCER

When we talk about the social process, women are usually forced to endure suffering, even more so when they are diagnosed with breast cancer, because their social and psychological context is affected due to the various feelings (PINHO *et a!,* 2007).

When a woman worries about her death, her psychological health is totally affected. It's at this point that she thinks about how her family will be, how she will cope, and even sometimes questions her faith, because she thinks that "God" at this point didn't care about her feelings or her duty to everyone.

From the moment they are diagnosed, many women end up isolating themselves from society and choose to go through the most difficult time of their lives alone, often because they are unable to express their feelings, turning it into a much worse pain than just what the disease could cause.

THEME: RIGHTS OF BREAST CANCER PATIENTS

Anyone who has cancer, regardless of the type, enjoys rights and benefits guaranteed by law, some of which are IPVA exemption, full withdrawal of FGTS, sickness benefit, among others (ROSA *etal.,* 2014).

Mammography is a woman's first right when it comes to breast cancer. It is an essential health right, because it is the preventive step that Brazilian public health so desperately wants for its population.

Breast cancer patients have the right to vocational rehabilitation, i.e. Social Security must re-educate and/or re-adapt so that the patient can return to work with dignity, which includes all ways to improve their quality of life while at work.

Sickness benefit is paid on a monthly basis as long as the patient is away from paid work for more than fifteen days, undergoing a medical examination and finding that they are unable to work; cancer patients must have contributed at least twelve months to receive this benefit. It stops being paid when the individual is deemed fit to return to their normal paid activities (ROSA *et a!,* 2014).

Retirement on the grounds of invalidity is when it is established by an expert that there is really no way of resuming paid activities, thus entering the retirement process (ROSA *et al.,* 2014).

Cancer patients are also exempt from income tax, IPTU (for cities that have this exemption law for cancer patients), IPVA and discounts on the purchase of new vehicles. They can withdraw all their available PIS and FGTS balances. In addition to having the option of paying off their home mortgage, provided they are unfit and the illness was acquired after the purchase contract was signed, they have this option due to the fact that the instalments also include an insurance policy that guarantees complete payment of their property. They also have the right to free transport so that they can get around to complete their treatment (ROSA *etal.,* 2014).

Brazilian Law No. 9797 of 1999 provides that women who have undergone total or partial mastectomy are entitled to reconstructive plastic surgery, and in the event of technical and medical conditions, the procedure can take place immediately after the cancer has been removed (BARRETO *et al.,* 2008; GALDINO *et a!,* 2017;' RODRIGUES *et al.,* 2017). It's a totally free procedure supported by SUS, but it does require an appointment so that everything can be done as desired by the patient.

CHAPTER 5

FINAL CONSIDERATIONS

Breast cancer affects women all over the world, with more than a million new cases every year. Its treatment varies greatly according to the tumour of each woman diagnosed.

One solution for curing this disease is mastectomy, which was the first medical surgical procedure capable of curing this pathology. It removes the affected breast, preventing it from spreading to other organs. However, the female breast has always been a highly valued part of the body, referring to values such as femininity and fertility. It can therefore be difficult for a woman to lose her breast. It's a situation that can lead to problems with self-esteem and acceptance of one's own body.

Analysing the themes made it possible to understand not only some aspects of the reality of women with neoplasia, but also their own perception of the moment they are facing. It's important to emphasise that each woman reacts to these situations according to a number of variables that relate to her life history, her social, economic and family context.

As you can see, there are two moments that women affected by cancer consider to be significant. The first moment is characterised by the discovery of cancer, which also involves diagnosis and treatment in which the battle to maintain life is very evident. Women begin to live daily with the possibility of death associated with the representations present in the social imaginary about breast cancer. In a second moment, which involves the post-surgical period, women resume their daily lives after overcoming the fear of death. The resumption of social relationships, leisure activities, work and family is when concerns about their own bodies arise.

The woman who has undergone treatment and a mastectomy has to realise that it was a procedure so that she could have the opportunity to live longer and rebuild herself in all biological and emotional aspects.

BIBLIOGRAPHICAL REFERENCES

ABRAHÃO, CM; FERRIAN, AM; GOMES, JR; LINO, AR; CRUZ, MRS. "Metaplastic carcinoma of the breast: the importance of anatomopathological confirmation". Rev. *Bras. Mastologia.* 2014; 24(2): 47-51. DOI: 10.5327/Z201400020004RBM "

ALMEIDA, RA. "The impact of mastectomy on women's lives". Rev. SBPH v.9 n.2 Rio de Janeiro dec. 2006. Available at : <http://pepsic.bvsalud.org/scielo.php?script=sci_arttext&pid=S1516-08582006000200007>. Accessed on: 29/08/2017.

AMERICAN CANCER SOCIETY. "Types of Breast Cancer. American Cancer Society medical information is copyrighted material. 2017. Available at: <https://www.cancer.org/cancer/breast-cancer/understanding-a-breast-cancer-

diagnosis/types-of-breast-cancer.html>. Accessed on: 08/08/2018.

AMERICAN CANCER SOCIETY. "Radiation for Breast Cancer. 2016. Available at :< https://www.google.com.br/search?q=https%2F%2Fwww.cancer.org%2Fcancer%2F breast-cancer%2Ftreatment%2Fradiation-for-breast-cancer.html&rlz=1C1VFKB_enBR797BR797&oq=https%2F%2Fwww.cancer.org%2F cancer%2Fbreast-cancer%2Ftreatment%2Fradiation-for-breast-cancer.html&aqs=chrome..69i57j69i58.951j0j4&sourceid=chrome&ie=UTF-8 >. Accessed on: 07/08/2018.

ARAB, C; DEMONICO, BB; CORREIA, CK; VILARINO, GT; ANDRADE, A. "Breast cancer and emotional reactions: a systematic review". *Rev. Baiana saúde pública',* 40 (2016). Available at: <http://pesquisa.bvsalud.org/portal/resource/pt/biblio- 876183>. Accessed 17/11/2017.

BARCELOS, MRB; VERENO FILHO, AL; CHAMBÔ FILHO, A; GUIMARÃES, RA; CINTRA, LC. "Intracystic Papillary Carcinoma of the Breast: Literature Review and Report of Two Cases". *Revista Brasileira de Cancerologia* - Volume 45 n°3 Jul/Aug/Sep 1999.

BARRETO, RAS; SUZUKI, K; LIMA, MA; MOREIRA, AA. "The information needs of mastectomised women subsidising nursing care". Revista Eletrónica de Enfermagem. 2008;10(1):110-123. Available at: < http://repositorio.bc.ufg. br/bitstream/ri/35/1/5460.pdf >. Accessed on: 25/09/2017.

BARROS, ACSD; BARBOSA, EM; GEBRIM, LH; *etal.* "Diagnosis and Treatment of Breast Cancer". Brazilian Society of Mastology. Brazilian Society of Cancerology. Brazilian Society of Pathology. Brazilian Federation of Gynaecology and Obstetrics. Guidelines Project. *Brazilian Medical Association and Federal Council of Medicine.* August 2001.

BOING, L; ARAÚJO, CCR; PEREIRA, GS; MORATELLI, J; BENNETI, M; BORGATTO, AF; BERGAMANN, A; GUIMARÃES, ACA. "Sitting time, body image and quality of life in women after breast cancer surgery". Rev Bras Med Esporte vol.23 no.5 São Paulo Sept./Oct. 2017. Available at:

<http://www.scielo.br/scielo.php?script=sci_arttext&pid=S1517-86922017000500366&lang=pt>. Accessed on: 17/08/2017.

BRAZIL. MINISTRY OF HEALTH. "ABC DO CÂNCER - Basic approaches to cancer control. National Cancer Institute (INCA). Rio de Janeiro. 2011.

BRAZIL. Ministry of Health. Health Care Secretariat. National Cancer Institute. Coordination of Prevention and Surveillance. Technical parameters for programming breast cancer early detection actions. Recommendations for state and municipal managers. Rio de Janeiro: Ministry of Health - INCA; 2006.

COMIN, FS; SANTOS, MA; SOUZA, LV. "Experiences and discourses of mastectomised women: negotiations and challenges of breast cancer". Estudos de Psicologia, 14(1), January-April/2009, 41-50. Available at: < http://www.scielo.br/pdf/epsic/v14n1/a06v14n1>. Accessed on: 17/08/2017.

FARIA, NC; FANGEL, LMV; ALMEIDA, AM; PRADO, MAS; CARLO, MMRP. "Psychosocial adjustment after mastectomy - a look at quality of life". Psic., Saúde & Doenças vol. 17 no.2 Lisboa Sep. 2016. Available at: <http://www.scielo.mec.pt/scielo.php?script=sci_arttext&pid=S1645-00862016000200008&lang=en>. Accessed on: 20/08/2017.

FRAZÃO, A; SKABA, MMFV. "Women with breast cancer: expressions of the social issue during neoadjuvant chemotherapy treatment". *Brazilian Journal of Cancerology.* 2013; 59(3): 427-435

GALDINO, AR; PEREIRA, LD; COSTA NETO, SB; BRANDÃO, CS; AMORIM, MHC. "Quality of life of mastectomised women enrolled in a rehabilitation programme". *Rev. Pesqui. Cuid. Fundam.* (Online); 9(2): 451-458, Apr-Jun. 2017. Available at: <http://pesquisa.bvsalud.org/portal/resource/pt/biblio-836362>. Accessed on: 29/08/2017.

HADDAD, CF. "Trastuzamab in breast cancer". Feminine. Feb-2010. Vol 38. No. 2. Available at: < http://files.bvs.br/upload/S/0100-7254/2010/v38n2/a001.pdf>. Accessed on 09/08/2018.

INCA. National Cancer Institute. Breast Cancer. 2018. Available at: <http://www2.inca.gov.br/wps/wcm/connect/tiposdecancer/site/home/mama>. Accessed on: 08/08/2018.

INCA. National Cancer Institute. Cancer incidence in Brazil. 2018. Available at: < http://www.inca.gov.br/estimativa/2018/>. Accessed on 09/08/2018.

JAMMAL, ML; MACHADO, ARM; RODRIGUES, LR. "Physiotherapy in the rehabilitation of women operated on for breast cancer". O *Mundo da Saúde São Paulo.* 2008; 32(4): 506-10.

MACHADO, MX; SOARES, DA; OLIVEIRA, SB. "Meanings of breast cancer for women in the context of chemotherapy treatment". Physis. 2017. Available at: <https://www.scielosp.org/scielo.php?script=sci_arttext&pid=S0103-73312017000300433&lang=pt>. Accessed on: 15/11/2017.

MAJEWSKI, JM; LOPES, ADF; DAVOGLIO, T; LEITE, JCC. "Quality of life in women who underwent mastectomy compared to those who underwent conservative surgery: a literature review". *Ciência & Saúde Coletiva,* 17(3):707-716, 2012. Available at :< http://www.scielo.br/pdf/csc/v17n3/v17n3a17.pdf>. Accessed on: 08/09/2017.

MATHEUS, VS; KESTELMAN, FP; CANELLA, EO; DJAHJAH, MCR; KOCH, HA. "Medullary carcinoma of the breast: anatomical and radiological correlation". *Radiol Bras* vol.41 no.6 São Paulo Nov./Dec. 2008. ISSN 1678-7099.

MENDES, K.D.S.; SILVEIRA, R.C.C.P.; GALVÃO, C.M. Integrative review: a research method for incorporating evidence in health and nursing. *Texto Contexto- Enferm.* v.17, n.4, 2008.

MOURA, FMJSP; SILVA, MG; OLIVEIRA, SC; MOURA, LJSP. "The feelings of post-mastectomised women". *Esc Anna Nery (impr.)* 2010 Jul-Sep; 14 (3): 477- 484.

NASCIMENTO, FB; PITTA, MGR; RÊGO, MJBM. "Analysing the main breast cancer diagnostic methods as drivers in the innovation process". Arq Med vol. 29 no. 6 Porto Dec. 2015. Available at:< http://www.scielo.mec.pt/scielo.php?script=sci_arttext&pid=S0871-34132015000600003>. Accessed on 09/08/2018.

OLIVEIRA, CF; SILVA, TS. "Invasive carcinoma of the breast: from diagnosis to surgical treatment". *Gynaecology Manual - Volume II.* Chapter 37. Pag 247- 288. ed. Permanyer, 2011. Available at: <http://www.fspog.com/fotos/editor2/cap_37.pdf>. Accessed 08/08/2018.

ONCOGUIA. The breast. Oncoguia Institute. 2014. Available at: < http://www.oncoguia.org.br/conteudo/a-mama/748/12/>. Accessed on: 03/08/2018.

ONCOGUIA. Types of Breast Cancer. Oncoguia Institute. 2014. Available at: < http://www.oncoguia.org.br/conteudo/tipos-de-cancer-de-mama/1382/34/>. Accessed on: 30/07/2018.

PINHO, LS; CAMPOS, ACS; FERNANDES, AFC; LOBO, SA. "Breast cancer: from discovery to recurrence of the disease". *Revista Eletrónica de Enfermagem.* 2007 Jan-Apr; 9(1): 154-165.

RBA. Rede Brasil Atual. RBA newsroom. Health and Science. "Sixty thousand women will be diagnosed with breast cancer this year". Mar/2018. Available at: < https://www.redebrasilatual.com.br/saude/2018/03/sem-prevencao-e-diagnostico- precoce-60-mil-mulheres-terao-diagnostico-de-cancer-de-mama>. Accessed on: 09/08/2018.

RITTO, MNG; BAPTISTA, CF; ALMEIDA, SMG; GIODARNO, MG; BRAGA, APF; OLIVEIRA, RPB. "Adenoid cystic carcinoma of the breast". *Rev. Bras. Mastologia',* 15 (3): 135-137, Sep. 2005. Illus.

RODRIGUES, NS; ORSINI, MRCA; MACHADO, AA; MONTIEL, JM; BARTHOLOMEU, D; TERTULIANO, IW. "Importance of psychological counselling for mastectomised women: review article". *ACM arch. Catarin. Med.*

46(1): 164-172 jan - mar 2017. Available at: < http://pesquisa.bvsalud.org/portal/resource/pt/biblio-847367 >. Accessed on: 24/09/2017.

ROSA, LFA; GIRARDON-PERLINI, NMO; STAMM, B; COUTO, MS; CARDOSO, AL; BIRK, NM. "Legal rights of people with cancer: knowledge of users of a public oncology service". Rev Enferm UFSM 2014 Oct/Dec; 4(4):771-783

SCLOWITZ, ML; MENEZES, AMB; GIGANTE, DP; TESSARO, S. "Conducts in the secondary prevention of breast cancer and associated factors". *Rev. Saúde Pública.* 2005; 39(3): 340-9.

TAVARES, JSC; TRAD, LAB. "Breast cancer coping strategies: a case study with families of mastectomised women". 2010. Available at: <http://www.repositorio.ufba. br:8080/ri/bitstream/ri/2358/1/repos2010.11 .pdf>. Accessed on: 07/09/2017.

VIEIRA, AV; TOIGO, FT. "BI-RADS Classification: Categorisation of 4,968 Mammograms". Radiol Bras vol.35 no.4 São Paulo July/aug. 2002. Available at: <http://www.scielo.br/scielo.php?script=sci_arttext&pid=S0100- 39842002000400005>. Accessed 08/08/2018.

VIAL, IL; FUENZALIDA RR; PIZARRO, FC; ROJAS, VO; VIAL, GL. "Prophylactic surgery in hereditary breast cancer syndrome". *Rev Chi! Cir* vol.68 no.6 Santiago dic. 2016. Available at : <http://www.scielo.cl/scielo.php?script=sci_arttext&pid=S0718-40262016000600013&lang=pt>. Accessed on: 20/11/2017.

XAVIER, D. "Breast cancer in Brazil". 2009. Available at: <https://www.webartigos.com/artigos/o-cancer-de-mama-no-brasil/16632/>. Accessed on 07/08/2018.

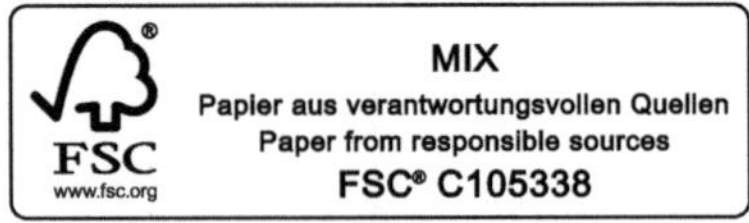

Printed by Books on Demand GmbH, Norderstedt / Germany